HEALTH POLICY A

EMERGING POLICIES
for
BIOMEDICAL RESEARCH

William N. Kelley
Marian Osterweis
Elaine R. Rubin
Editors

ASSOCIATION OF ACADEMIC HEALTH CENTERS

T he Association of Academic Health Centers (AHC) is a national, nonprofit organization comprising more than 100 institutional members in the United States and Canada that are the health complexes of the nation's major universities. Academic health centers consist of an allopathic or osteopathic school of medicine, at least one other health professions school or program, and one or more teaching hospitals. These institutions are the nation's primary resources for education in the health professions, biomedical and health services research, and many aspects of patient care services.

The AHC seeks to influence public dialogue on significant health and science policy issues, to advance education for health professionals, to promote biomedical and health services research, and to enhance patient care.

The views expressed in this book are those of its authors and do not necessarily represent the views of the Board of Directors of the Association of Academic Health Centers or the membership at large.

Copyright 1993 by the Association of Academic Health Centers
All rights reserved. Published 1993
Printed in the United States of America
Library of Congress Catalog Card Number: 93-071077
ISBN 1-879694-06-9
ISSN 1056-2389

Copies of this book may be purchased from:
Association of Academic Health Centers
1400 Sixteenth Street, NW, Suite 410
Washington, DC 20036
202/265-9600 Fax: 202/265-7514
Price: $20.00 plus $3.00 postage and handling

Design and Production: Fletcher Design, Washington, DC

This book is printed on recycled paper.

Contents

Preface

The unprecedented ascent of the biomedical sciences in the United States since World War II has changed not only the fabric of American society but also the lives of people throughout the world. The products of research, which run the gamut from individual discoveries to corporate biotechnology enterprises, greatly contributed to securing the United States as a world power.

The policies of growth and expansion spawned success; the nation can point with pride to the many benefits of its investment in science, including national research facilities, international recognition, advances in medicine and public health, and technological breakthroughs that were translated into industrial applications and consumer products. Less apparent but no less important are the untold benefits that come from increased employment, vast economic development, an array of new services, improved productivity, and finally, a heightened sense of public understanding of and appreciation for science.

At the same time, this very progress has been a major factor in creating controversy and concern about the nature and direction of science. The frontiers of knowledge have expanded at an unimagined pace: In the biomedical sciences a revolution has occurred. The monumental results of that revolution are only now being fully translated into improving health care.

The speed of discovery has accelerated and the time from discovery to industrial application has shortened. This rapid pace has transformed the scientific enterprise and created a different set of societal expectations about the goals and products of research. New collaborative and entrepreneurial arrangements have also developed to enhance the conduct of research and to speed the commercialization process. Many of the current problems and dilemmas, whether created in the laboratories, the halls of Congress, or the courts of law, have resulted from the very newness of science that often forces the development of policies on issues never before recognized or thought possible.

While society has reaped extraordinary benefits from the discoveries and applications of biomedical research, doubts have emerged about the societal commitment to research and the advance of scientific knowledge, the appropriate nature of scientific inquiry, the integrity of researchers, the selection of priorities and the allocation of funds, the appropriate applications of scientific discoveries, the legal and ethical implications of the use of scientific information, and the roles and responsibilities of government, industry, and the academic community.

Our society approaches the next century in a state of flux and uncertainty. While the public recognizes that scientific progress ensures achievement in every aspect of American life and culture, the goals, resources, attitudes, and commitments of individuals, institutions, and the public are under scrutiny. Tensions and turmoil have surfaced to threaten the scientific enterprise in the 1990s as new science coupled with shifting political and educational paradigms challenge the public policy arena.

Biomedical research policy was selected as the theme for this third volume of the health policy series published by the Association of Academic Health Centers (AHC). The major breakthroughs during the 1960s and 1970s, which made recombinant DNA technology possible, accelerated the pace of discoveries to prevent, treat, and cure disease and significantly heightened awareness about the magnitude and power of the biomedical sciences. Physics and engineering, which for many people constituted "science," were no longer the sole determinants of science policy related to national security or economic growth.

This book is significant and timely for it addresses public policy and the challenging and controversial scientific issues that confront decision makers in the 1990s. It not only highlights the current environment for policymaking but also focuses on the forces of change, the emerging issues, and the unresolved problems that contribute to the development and implementation of public policy.

A literature that deals exclusively with the development and analysis of biomedical research policy is difficult to delineate. What does emerge is a literature of specifics—resource allocation issues, legislative acts, interest group politics, legal controversies, or particular scientific discoveries. A coherent set of writings on biomedical science policy was not forthcoming from the journals and reports dedicated to science.

Therefore, we view this publication as a beginning contribution to the construction of a literature dedicated to a broad vision of biomedical science policy. The origins of public policy are often difficult to determine. Causes, motivations, and influences can often never fully be known. At all levels of decisionmaking, a definite course or method of action is not always evident, and conditions that might guide or determine present or future decisions may be variously understood or misunderstood. An all-embracing plan, general goals, or acceptable procedures may be deemed prudent or totally unwise at any point in time.

This book attempts to fill the void in policy literature with perhaps the first compilation and categorization of published articles and reports from 1991 and 1992 that develop questions related to biomedical research policy. A unique format of abstracts, excerpts and commentaries makes the book a useful reference tool and handy policy handbook.

From the funding of individual investigators to the concern for globalization and technology development, this book attempts to outline the issues, define the priorities, analyze the problems, highlight the conflicts, and present new perspectives on policy.

The opening chapter describes the philosophical basis for public support for the biomedical research enterprise and details the incredible history of the establishment of the National Institutes of Health (NIH).

The eleven chapters that follow provide the reader with abstracts and excerpts of selected articles and reports along with short commentaries on issues ranging from societal goals to scientific publications. The commentaries were written by members of the AHC

Task Force on Science Policy and other AHC members who have been examining science policy questions for several years.

The AHC members, chief executive officers of the nation's academic health centers, offer a broad perspective on the biomedical research enterprise, which is an integral part of their institutions. The academic health centers, the health complexes of the major universities across the country, are dedicated to education of health professionals and training of biomedical research scientists, to the conduct of research in the biomedical sciences, and to the provision of health care services. The commentators do not necessarily seek to resolve debates and dilemmas but rather to offer insight and analysis, often from a personal or institutional perspective, of the complex interface between science and society. We have excluded issues relating to the education and training of scientists because these human resource questions will be the focus of next year's health policy annual.

A critical thread throughout the work is America's investment in fundamental research and the partnership between the government and the academic community. The university, which has been at the core of the scientific enterprise of the United States for more than 50 years, has been the key to that relationship.

Our public policies have made universities the sites not only for the conduct of research but also the education and training of the next generation of scientists. As the developers of science, universities have been accepted and celebrated as national resources and keys to our national survival.

Of great significance is the marriage that took place in the 1980s between the profit orientation of industry and the knowledge quest of the university. Although encouraged by public policies, attitudes changed as universities turned to industry for additional basic research support. Scientists were encouraged to commercialize their discoveries and to merge the basic and applied research cultures. Academic institutions established relationships with industry. Venture capitalists courted universities, and state and local governments perceived the universities as resources for creating economic development.

The university-industrial relationship has been successful, giving rise to unimagined advances, most notably in molecular biology and genetic engineering. These advances resulted in new technology and biological products that today are accepted as invaluable in the diagnosis and treatment of illness and disease.

Yet, the fundamental goals and values of the universities, these trusted institutions that have been committed to the pursuit of new knowledge, are now under attack. Of particular concern to universities are the ability to manage research, the integrity of research, the nature of scientific misconduct in research, and the costs that the public should bear to support biomedical research.

On many issues there is no consensus. For many people, the basic principles of biomedical research are at issue with the future of science dependent on the rationale that policymakers choose to espouse in funding scientific investigation. In this era of federal budget deficits and general fiscal constraint, policymakers are shifting and redefining the priorities for public investment. There is fear that short-term visions about national scientific resources, economic development, or cost containment are driving public policy. Such a trend, many argue, can do irreparable harm to the scientific enterprise.

The need to support fundamental research is central to the argument for long-term strategies. The basis for progess for generations has been fundamental science and the ability of the scientific mind to freely examine, observe, and study. This foundation has also provided the capability to conduct research in a range of new interdisciplinary areas.

The human genome project, for example, may symbolize the success that can be achieved when unfettered science provides the environment for the convergence of so many disciplines and technologies. This international effort to map and sequence the human genome is a product of fundamental scientific advances in many fields, including genetics, molecular biology, and biotechnology. The project too shows the controversies of progress; while there is general agreement that the products of the project will revolutionize medicine, there is also concern about the many, yet-to-be answered ethical, legal, and social questions.

The politics of public policy are revealed in the articles dedicated to the development of the strategic plan for the NIH. Called "A Strategic Vision" in its final version, the plan highlights the importance of the policymaking process as well as the conflict that can result from redefining priorities, whether they be for the government's research institutes or the departments of a particular university.

Many people perceived the planning process as closed; constituents were not properly consulted; time was short; public meetings were mismanaged, indeed, orchestrated, according to some observers. In short, politics and packaging were said by some to overshadow science and sensibility. Was the document a blueprint for the future—a strategic vision—or was it an agenda for government-directed research? Was the scientific enterprise to be micromanaged from the nation's capital? Was science merely a tool to enhance America's economic competitiveness? Was basic research to be sacrificed to financial necessity or the politics of health care reform? Or was the plan a carefully conceived mechanism to stimulate continued congressional support and funding and to ensure an open pipeline between advances in fundamental science and the improved health of the public? These questions will continue to be debated as the NIH seeks to implement the plan.

Competing values and outlooks can also become sources of conflict when new areas of research are opened, such as the Women's Health Initiative at the NIH, or new priorities for funding are established as occurred with AIDS research.

The emergence of new diseases such as AIDS also demonstrates the power of the public to influence policy decisions. Public opinion and public interest groups may play an increasingly important role in policymaking as we move toward the 21st Century. In this regard, scientists are being forced to expand their horizons beyond the laboratories and to educate and inform the public about all aspects of the research environment. In such efforts, the media will remain a critical point of contact on issues of science and technology and one that needs to be reckoned with.

Clearly, difficult choices lie ahead. Individuals and institutions may need to adapt or to reorganize to survive these changing times. The need for adequate information, careful analysis, public education, and solid outcomes will become even more critical to decision-making at all levels. We hope this book will contribute to the current dialogue and suggest new areas of discussion. And too, it may show the need to develop greater consensus on particular issues so that the United States can maintain its leadership and international preeminence.

We would like to thank the members of the Editorial Advisory Board for their invaluable assistance in recommending pieces for inclusion in this publication. A special thanks also goes to Joan Durgin, AHC administrative assistant, for her excellent work in typing the manuscript and helping to prepare it for publication.

William N. Kelley
Marian Osterweis
Elaine R. Rubin
Editors

Editorial Advisory Board

Others

Lawrence K. Altman, M.D.
Medical Correspondent
The New York Times

Katherine Bick, M.D.
Scientific Liaison USA
Centro Studio Multicentrico
  Italiano sulla Demenza

Roger J. Bulger, M.D.
President
Association of Academic Health
  Centers

Ruth Bulger, Ph.D.
Director, Division on Health
  Sciences Policy
Institute of Medicine
National Academy of Sciences

Rosemary Chalk
Study Director
Commission on Behavioral and
  Social Sciences and Education
National Academy of Sciences

Henry R. Desmarais, M.D., M.P.A.
Principal
Health Policy Alternatives, Inc.

Jack C. Ebeler
Principal
Health Policy Alternatives, Inc.

Alfred P. Fishman, M.D.
William Maul Measey Professor of
  Medicine
and Chairman, Department of
  Rehabilitation Medicine
Hospital of the University of
  Pennsylvania

Donald S. Fredrickson, M.D.
Consultant and
Former Director
National Institutes of Health

Roger C. Herdman, M.D.
Assistant Director
Health and Life Sciences Division
Office of Technology Assessment

Douglas E. Kelly, Ph.D.
Associate Vice President
Division of Biomedical Research
Association of American Medical
  Colleges

Elaine L. Larson, R.N., Ph.D.
Dean, School of Nursing
Georgetown University and
*AHC Scholar in Academic
  Administration & Health Policy*

Richard A. Lauderbaugh, J.D.
Principal
Health Policy Alternatives, Inc.

Joshua Lederberg, Ph.D.
University Professor
The Rockefeller University

Thomas E. Malone, Ph.D.
Vice President, Division of
  Biomedical Research
Association of American Medical
  Colleges

Stephen M. Merz
Research Assistant
Association of Academic Health
  Centers

Barbara Mishkin, J.D.
Hogan & Hartson

Rodney W. Nichols
Chief Executive Officer
New York Academy of Sciences

Gilbert S. Omenn, M.D., Ph.D.
Dean, School of Public Health
    and
Community Medicine
Professor of Medicine and of
    Environmental Health
University of Washington

Marian Osterweis, Ph.D.
Vice President
Association of Academic Health
    Centers

Frederick C. Robbins, M.D.
University Professor and Dean
    Emeritus
School of Medicine
Case Western Reserve University

Elaine R. Rubin, Ph.D.
Program Associate
Association of Academic Health
    Centers

Albert Teich
Director, Science and Policy
    Programs
American Association for the
    Advancement of Science

Contributors

Carol A. Aschenbrener, M.D., is chancellor of the University of Nebraska Medical Center.

Jack D. Barchas, M.D., is dean for research development and dean for neuroscience of the School of Medicine at the University of California, Los Angeles.

Isaac D. Barchas is a Century Fellow in the Committee on Social Thought of the University of Chicago.

David A. Blake, Ph.D., is senior associate dean of the School of Medicine of The Johns Hopkins University.

Roger J. Bulger, M.D., is president of the Association of Academic Health Centers.

David R. Challoner, M.D., is vice president for health affairs of the University of Florida.

Neil S. Cherniack, M.D., is vice president for medical affairs and dean of the School of Medicine at Case Western Reserve University.

Leslie Cutler, D.D.S., Ph.D., is interim vice president and interim provost for health affairs, and interim executive director of the University of Connecticut Health Center.

James E. Dalen, M.D., is vice provost for health sciences and dean of the School of Medicine at the University of Arizona.

F. Daniel Davis is director of planning & communications at the Georgetown University Medical Center.

Thomas Detre, M.D., is senior vice chancellor for health sciences of the University of Pittsburgh.

Donald S. Fredrickson, M.D., is a consultant and former director of the National Institutes of Health.

John F. Griffith, M.D., is executive vice president for health sciences, director of the medical center and executive dean of the medical school of the Georgetown University Medical Center.

Donald C. Harrison, M.D., is senior vice president and provost for health education of the University of Cincinnati Medical Center.

H. Garland Hershey, Jr., D.D.S., is vice chancellor for health affairs and vice provost of the university of The University of North Carolina at Chapel Hill.

Michael E. Johns, M.D., is dean of the medical faculty and vice president for medicine at The Johns Hopkins University.

William N. Kelley, M.D., is executive vice president for the medical center and dean of the School of Medicine at The University of Pennsylvania.

David Korn, M.D., is vice president and dean of the School of Medicine at the Stanford University Medical Center.

Marian Osterweis, Ph.D., is vice president of the Association of Academic Health Centers.

Cynthia Maurer-Sutton, C.P.A., M.B.A., is associate executive vice president for venture and industry relationships at the School of Medicine of the University of Pennsylvania.

Herbert Pardes, M.D., is vice president for health sciences and dean of the faculty of the College of Physicians & Surgeons at Columbia University.

William A. Peck, M.D., is vice chancellor for medical affairs and dean of the School of Medicine at the Washington University Medical Center.

Elaine R. Rubin, Ph.D., is program associate of the Association of Academic Health Centers.

Ralph Snyderman, M.D., is chancellor for health affairs and dean of the School of Medicine at the Duke University Medical Center.

Jay H. Stein, M.D., is senior vice president and provost of the Oklahoma City Campus of the University of Oklahoma.

Manuel Tzagournis, M.D., is vice president for health services and dean of the College of Medicine at The Ohio State University.

James A. Zimble, M.D., is president of the Uniformed Services University of the Health Sciences.

CHAPTER I

Biomedical Science and the Culture Warp

Donald S. Fredrickson

One winter's night in Helsinki during the 1970s, I was guest of honor at a dinner in the American Embassy for a group of distinguished Finnish academicians. The ambassador, under the nom de théâtre of Mark Evans, had been producer and host of a popular television talk show in Washington. After dinner, brandy in hand, I found myself responding to the announcement of the master of ceremonies that I was going to explain how medical science was supported in the U.S. by the National Institutes of Health.

My discourse wandered from intramural research to study sections and finally to public participation in the governance of science. I noted that the national advisory councils are one example of such public participation. I also pointed to the national commissions that were devoted to the study of specific diseases such as diabetes and arthritis. These were established by congressional orders and had emerged from concerns of citizens suffering from those diseases. Finally, I outlined the congressional hearings on the annual appropriation for the NIH. As I described how the congressmen would later invite testimony from lay witnesses about our performances, the president of the Finnish Academy of Sciences abruptly rose from his seat. He could not imagine such public interference in the conduct of science in Finland, nor for that matter, in any other European society. All the other listeners seemed to share his judgment. There was a moment of silence as I groped about for a metaphor to save the situation. Pointing at one of the tapestries on the embassy wall, I likened the acquisition and organization of wisdom to weaving. Consider the gathering of threads of knowledge as the *weft*, I suggested, and the orthogonal *warp* threads stretched in the loom as essential support for making the fabric. In my country, I continued, the strength of this warp and the tension upon it came from many sources, by no means limited to scientists. Our scientific research therefore was woven on a *culture warp*, I ended, insisting that, despite the great number of hands involved in the setting of the loom, production was actually amplified and accelerated.

A distinguished task force of the Carnegie Commission on Science, Technology, and Government concerned with long-term federal science and technology goals has recently issued a thoughtful report.[1] The report's principal recommendation is the creation of a forum of "individuals from industry, academia, nongovernmental organizations, and the interested public to explore and seek consensus on long-term [societal] S&T goals...." The National Academy of Sciences (NAS) is suggested as a possible venue. This proposal for obtaining better advice on a rational deployment of federal support addresses a dilemma as old as the republic: that is, there is no constitutional prescription specifically linking science *per se* to the public purse. By opening with the traditional reference to Vannevar Bush's *Science: The Endless Frontier*,[2] the Carnegie report reminds me of Bush's earlier experience in convening a forum of the elite of industry, academia, and researchers to design a new departure in federal policy toward science. Bush's report was written almost 50 years ago toward the end of World War II. His plan for creating a single agency to underwrite basic research in the private sector with federal funds eventually resulted in the creation of the National Science Foundation. Bush's original design, however, was upset and materially changed by unforeseen interventions that illustrated the limitations of any one group—however expert and well-meaning— in defining societal goals. Although this history has been several times told,[3-6] it merits retelling. The generation that remembers well the roots of today's system of support for biomedical research—and the accompanying growth of our country's academic institutions to their present size and research capacity—is becoming emeritus. This tale also contains instruction on the nature, complexity, and durability of the culture warp of biomedical science.

SCIENCE FOR WAR

The Establishment of the OSRD (1941)

Vannevar Bush was a Yankee of remarkable accomplishments. He was an inventor (the Bush differential analyzer enabled the start of modern computer analysis), an educator (dean of engineering at MIT), and scientific leader (president of the Carnegie Institution of Washington and director of the Office of Scientific Research and Development (OSRD) (1941-1946)). In 1940 when war had broken out in Europe, Bush discussed with some of his friends, including Karl Compton, James Bryant Conant, and Frank Jewett, the need to mobilize American science for preparedness in the event the country was drawn into the hostilities. These men first convinced President Roosevelt and Congress to form a National Defense Research Committee (NRDC). This committee was established on July 2, 1940, and was chaired initially by Bush.[7] In June 1941, at Bush's insistence, the President issued an executive order establishing the OSRD to coordinate and supervise all research related to the national defense; Bush was named as director.[8] The NRDC became a subdivision of the OSRD, concerned with weapons development, and Conant became the director. Keeping his office in the Carnegie headquarters, Bush looked to the National Academy of Sciences

(NAS) and the National Research Council (NRC) to assist in the task of helping to select scientists or laboratories for projects with very specific objectives and which were to be supported by contract. The import and nature of some of the research involved can be judged by the presentation of the Atomic Pioneers Award to Bush, Conant, and General Leslie Groves by President Nixon in 1970.

Committee on Medical Research. Research in medicine was one of the high wartime priorities. The Germans had cornered the quinine supply, and new antimalarials had to be found. With only sulfonamides to treat infections, new chemotherapeutic agents were needed. Many other problems had to be tackled, such as improving the treatment of shock, and methods of transfusion, augmenting supplies of plasma and other blood products, understanding the physiology of high altitude aviation, motion sickness, and anoxia, and even developing new kinds of clothing.

In his memoirs,[9] Bush recalled that he had felt then that "he had nothing to do with medical research, and did not want to have...." However, as Presidential Counselor Judge Samuel Rosenman prepared the order setting up the OSRD, the Committee on Medical Research (CMR) was added after the president, weary of an office full of medical organizations each demanding to set up a medical research committee, ordered that "he wanted this medical show put under Bush and he didn't want to hear a damn thing more about it."[9] Bush then established the CMR on his own terms. He insisted that the CMR have strong attachment to the Division of Medical Services of the National Research Council (DMS-NRC), even basing it in the NAS building on Constitution Avenue. The more than forty committees and subcommittees of the DMS soon began to function as "study sections."[8] DMS members sometimes initiated proposals, outsiders initiated others. DMS reviewed each proposal and sent them to CMR with a recommendation. CMR in turn sent its own recommendations up to OSRD, where Bush's signature on the folio indicated final approval. The contracts tended to be categorical, with highly specific objectives. Their duration was short, sometimes for six months, and never for more than a year before review for possible renewal. The committees of the DMS were populated by high-level academics, including members of the NAS, and many elite clinician advisors, about one-third of whom were members of the "Old Turks," the Association of American Physicians.[10]   The chairman of the DMS, Lewis Weed, a professor of anatomy at Johns Hopkins Medical School, wanted to head the CMR, but Bush wanted a scientist of stature with impeccable qualifications. He personally picked A. Newton Richards, professor of pharmacology, vice president for medical affairs of the University of Pennsylvania Medical School, and a pioneer in micropuncture studies of the kidney.[9] Bush later summed up his selection: "It was a fortunate choice...I concluded that, of all the able men I've known, [Richards] was the most fully respected, yes, the most beloved by his colleagues and by everybody who knew him."[6]

The members of the CMR were seven: one each designated by the secretary of war, the secretary of the navy, and the head of the Federal Security Agency (then the parent agency of the Public Health Service), and four civilians appointed by the President. The latter were Chairman Richards,   A. R. Dochez, chairman of bacteriology at Columbia College of Physicians & Surgeons, A. Baird Hastings, professor of biochemistry at Harvard Medical School, and Professor Weed. Surgeon General Thomas Parran designated the director of NIH to fill his chair. Initially this was Lewis R. Thompson, who was followed in 1942 by Rolla E. (Gene) Dyer. Over its life, the CMR dispensed $24 million in some 600 contracts to 133 universities, foundations, and industrial laboratories, involving the research of over 1500 doctorates and 4000 laboratory personnel.[7]

The Dismantling of the OSRD (1944-45)

Bush had always believed that OSRD must go out of business as soon as the war was won. The exigencies of war were one thing, but like many of his contemporaries, Bush appears to also have had some deep-seated misgivings about government support of science in peacetime. At Cold Spring Harbor in 1960, before an audience at a dedication of a new laboratory building, Bush articulated the Carnegie Institution's resistance to accepting government support and described his fears that government subsidies would result in federal control over individual scientific efforts.[11] By August 1944, Bush was certain that he would like to see OSRD wind down as soon as the course of the war permitted and he let this be known to his advisory committees and presented the President with a program for the termination of OSRD. There was movement among the leaders of the armed services to maintain a capability for military research. Secretary of War Stimson favored the NAS's assuming responsibility for a Research Board for National Security to continue contracts for defense science. However, because of the NAS desire to protect its independent status and negative reaction from elsewhere in government, nothing came of this.

The CMR was informed as early as August 3 of Bush's demobilization decision and discussed at length its implications during its next meeting on August 17. The navy representative said that his service would not be able to take over any war research contracts. The surgeon general of the army and Dyer of the Public Health Service felt that the CMR should continue to the end of the war. Because, as we shall see later, the Public Health Service had earlier in 1944 received new research authority, Dyer also stated that the Public Health Service would have no legal problem in continuing projects appropriate to its functioning.[12]

Throughout the next twelve months, CMR sporadically requested further instruction on demobilization, and Bush from time to time assured Richards that OSRD and CMR were going to close but left the fate of the contracts uncertain. The ambiguity of the situation was suddenly increased in November by a fateful communication to Bush from the President.

The Roosevelt Letter of November 17, 1944

The President's letter to Vannevar Bush requested answers to four questions. The first was how the scientific achievements of the OSRD during the war could be called to the attention of the public. The fourth requested plans for increasing the number of research workers. But the two others that thereafter received the most attention asked how federal support for scientific research in public and private institutions—in medicine, on the one hand, and in the rest of science, on the other—might be continued in peacetime, a radical reversal of longtime government policy.[13]

Before turning to the answers and the drama of their development, one should pause to wonder why Franklin Roosevelt had come to write such a letter to Bush. Roosevelt was not hostile to science, but did not possess any discernible science policy. In addition, he had just been through his fourth presidential election and was bearing a crushing burden of running a war and planning for peace. Historians have tended to shy away from one available explanation. In a 1960 biography of Albert Lasker, John Gunther wrote that Mrs. Mary Lasker, just commencing her lifelong advocacy of government support for medical research in 1944, sent a note to FDR requesting the government to consider continuing medical research in peacetime. The letter went to the President through Anna Rosenberg, a member of the War Mobilization Advisory Board who had an office in the East Wing of the White House. The President is said to have then passed it on to Judge Rosenman, who in turn drafted the note to Bush.[14] In 1961 Calvin Baldwin, a former NIH colleague of mine, while doing research at Harvard on the origins of NIH, wrote a letter to Judge Rosenman, asking him about the authenticity of this story. The judge replied that he knew "nothing at all, one way or another..." about Gunther's reference.[15] This reply, along with a request for her recollections, was sent to Mrs. Rosenberg. It elicited a prompt letter in reply:

> John Gunther's reference ... as to how the National Institutes of Health came about is completely correct. I remember clearly this incident because I often thought about how the Institutes grew and became so important....Judge Rosenman did so many things at that time that he may not recall this particular letter, but I distinctly remember it.[16]

In his authoritative source on the origin of the National Science Foundation, J. Merton England has sifted the other evidence indicating that sources closer to Bush were at least also involved.[17] Carroll Wilson, an OSRD administrator, responded to a series of queries on the subject that "Bush did not write it [FDR's letter] nor did he ask for it, but he had the opportunity to see it before it was sent and made some suggestions which were incorporated." England further noted that "at least there is evidence that the letter came from outside the OSRD" and suggests a prominent possibility as Oscar Cox, a lawyer who had worked with Bush on setting up the NDRC and OSRD. Other sources indicate Bush met with Cox and the OSRD general counsel concerning the draft letter.

Whatever his involvement and personal opinions on several of the questions in the letter, Bush was a loyal public servant and a superb organizer. He quickly mobilized four teams of advisers and widely canvassed his powerful friends to help him frame answers for the President.

The Bowman Committee. Bush first turned to Isaiah Bowman to organize a committee to answer the President's broadest (third) question. Bowman, a geographer and member of the scientific elite, was president of The Johns Hopkins University as well as vice president of the NAS. An advocate of government support of science, Bowman had been chairman of the NRC during Roosevelt's first term. In an effort to stimulate federal subsidy of research, he had been instrumental in inducing FDR to form a Science Advisory Board (SAB). The short-lived SAB (1933-35), chaired by Karl Compton of MIT, was a chimeric creature of the NAS and a source of great controversy within the NAS because FDR had blithely overridden the NAS hard-won and jealously guarded prerogative to appoint its own committees.[18] As we shall see later, the SAB also became a vehicle for conveying an early pitch for more funding for the Public Health Service.

Third: What can the Government do now and in the future to aid research activities by public and private organizations. . .?[13]

The membership of the blue-ribbon Bowman Committee included at least two distinguished researchers, the inventor and industrialist Edwin Land and physicist I. I. Rabi, then at MIT. Seven members were deans or presidents from the galaxy of research universities. Industry was further represented by the director of Bell Laboratories and the chairmen of Standard Oil of Indiana and Dewey and Almay Chemicals. Also among the members were one or two government officials, including the director of the U.S. Geological Survey. There were no biomedical people aboard and, at its first meeting, the Bowman Committee noted that *clinical* medicine—subject of a direct presidential question—was assigned to another committee. The members set aside the social sciences as "to be handled as a special issue" and elected to confine themselves to peacetime research in the natural sciences, agriculture, and engineering in academic and nonprofit institutions.[19]

The final report of the committee—included as one of the main sections of Bush's report—provided a thoughtful and extensive assessment of the state of research in the U.S. during the depression of the 1930s.[2,18] It noted that, while industrial research had survived well and was continually increasing, the growth rate of private sources of financial support for nonprofit institutions had gone into a serious decline. Such sources included the Rockefeller and Carnegie foundations and their related funds that had accounted for much of the growth of the major research universities since the turn of the century and also had established two great nonprofit research institutes, the Rockefeller Institute and the Carnegie Institution. Over the decade of the 1930s, expenditures for research by colleges and universities had risen feebly, from only $21 million in 1930 to $41 million in 1940, while expenditures by nonprofit research institutes had actually fallen from $5.2 million in 1930 to $4.5 million in 1940. There was a sense of frustration, perhaps particularly among researchers in many of the natural sciences. The committee observed that medical research had been able to attract more private support than any other discipline and that it was only the American medical schools that could compete with the great European universities in both fundamental as well as practical or applied research.

The Bowman Committee found the temptation of peacetime government support to be a source of great anxiety, largely centering around the fear that federal aid would mean the imposition of federal control.

> It is the firm conviction of the Committee that centralized control of research by any small group of persons would be disastrous; if this small group were backed by the power and the prestige of the federal government and open to political influence, it would be catastrophic...[18]

The possibility that scientific freedom could thus be corrupted was accompanied by worry that federal aid might drive away the existing sources of funds, that private endowments might cease, the great foundations might turn to other fields, and states might reduce support given their large institutions. In the end, however, the pluses outweighed the negatives. The Bowman Committee members swallowed their fears and recommended that a National Research Foundation (NRF) be created under conditions that would minimize the perceived hazards. It would have to be governed by a board of scientists and their sympathizers, who would choose—and control—a compliant federal director.[18]

The Medical Advisory Committee

A day after receiving the President's letter, Bush informed Richards that he felt the CMR was overburdened and that he needed to get other opinions to help him answer the President's second question.[20] Bush asked the CMR to give him a list of possible advisers, which it worked assiduously to assemble. After the CMR had compiled a primary list of ten, it drew up a list of 150 more experts who might advise Bush. When this was done, someone, perhaps as an afterthought, advanced a resolution to the effect that, if a federal employee were included, it should be Gene Dyer. No sooner did this pass when the army and the navy representatives complained that should one service be included, all should be.[21] It was then decided that only names of civilians would be forwarded.

Second: With particular reference to the war of science against disease, what can be done now to organize a program for continuing. . .the work which has been done in medicine and related sciences?[13]

Within a few days, Bush wrote Walter Palmer, Bard professor of medicine at Columbia, and Homer Smith, professor of physiology at NYU,[22] requesting them to be chair and secretary, respectively, of his Medical Advisory Committee (MAC). The other members Bush chose were equally well-known academicians: William B. Castle, Edward A. Doisy, Ernest Goodpasture, Alton Ochsner, Linus Pauling, Kenneth B. Turner, and James J. Waring. Two invitees, Arthur Bloomfield and H. S. Gasser, declined. The advisers, who included five members of the NAS, a Nobel

Laureate (Doisy, for physiology or medicine in 1943), and one future Laureate (Pauling, for chemistry in 1954), were as blue-ribbon as the Bowman Committee and included more working scientists. Bush then wrote Richards to inform him of what he had done and reminded him,"it is well understood that OSRD and CMR go out of existence at the end of the war."[23] At the same time, however, CMR instructed division chiefs to present proposals to run beyond June 30, 1945.[8]

Not everyone believed that the opinions of the MAC would be useful. Bush's friend Frank Jewett, an industrial engineer of distinction and director of Bell Laboratories, was president of the NAS between 1939 and 1946, and he offered Bush the following candid opinion:

> If medical science is going to struggle with each one of these [diseases] as it takes the center of the stage (as I assume it will) its problems will exist forever. As fast as one specific thing is conquered another will crop up... as in the case of medicine, it seems to me questionable if a 'must' case for Federal support can be sustained as the only solution.[24]

On March 8, 1945, the first plenary meeting of the advisers gathered in Bush's office in Washington.[25] Homer Smith had already tipped the hand of the MAC in a letter to Bush.[26] Walter Palmer nevertheless read a prospectus written by Turner that gave the MAC opinion as unanimously favoring a separate agency for medical research, something on the lines of the British Medical Research Council (MRC). The MAC predilection for the British MRC as a model was understandable but perhaps only partially on target.[27,28] On the plus side was the fact that this medical science agency was relatively venerable (having been established in 1911) and from the first was operating with an absolute minimum of government interference. The highly university-oriented MAC members did not appear to realize, however, that a high proportion of MRC funds have always been committed to a large intramural program, which included The National Institute for Medical Research and a cadre of full-time employees in laboratories located at universities, but independent of them, such as the celebrated Molecular Biology Laboratory at Cambridge.

Bush, much displeased by this threat of insurrection, asked the MAC members if they had contacted the Public Health Service (PHS), since the interrelationship of such a new body and the PHS would have to be clear in order for Congress to go along with it.[24] Palmer and Smith indicated that their view had been endorsed by 350 representatives of 75 of the nation's medical schools, research institutions, pharmaceutical industries, and philanthropic foundations. Bush's staff, however, backed him up with a barrage of interoffice memos harshly criticizing the MAC position;[29] the Director's disapproval continued to trickle down to the drafters through Bush confidantes in New York who were assigned to help with the completion of the MAC report. The final revision of this document, submitted to Bush on April 15, was accompanied by a letter from Palmer that stated, "it becomes more and more evident to us in New York that our recommendations for an independent agency may be too idealistic and impractical..."[30] The final version of the MAC report that is published with the Bush Report nevertheless still contains the separatist views. Bush ignored the proposal and insisted that medical research would be retained in the new agency he had in mind. However, a number of the lyrical phrases about the achievements and promise of medical research in the MAC report were selected by Bush as part of the text of the body of *Science: the Endless Frontier.* The full MAC report, like the extensive reports of the Bowman Committee and the committee on scientific manpower (headed by Henry Allen Moe), was included in the appendices.

The Designs for the Purse
Who Should Run It? In seeking to immunize the new research agency from noxious influences of government management, the Bowman Committee specified that the new autonomous and independent body to be created by Congress should be "composed of men of the highest integrity, ability and experience, and with thorough understanding of the problems of science." They were to be "empowered to give sustained, far-sighted assistance to science with some form of assurance of continuing support." The Bowman Committee also recommended the establishment of a National Science Board to

concern itself with a global surveillance and rationalization of government support of science, a need that the Carnegie Commission has so lately readdressed in its 1992 report.[1] The MAC recommended that its National Federation of Medical Research should be administered by a board of trustees appointed by the President, with Senate confirmation, and a technical board of experts with aides and committees to oversee distribution and watch how the money was used. Everyone feared a strong administrator and demanded a passive one, beholden to the board.

How to Give Away the Money. The Bowman Committee and the MAC converged on one recommendation. The bulk of the funds was to be given to the universities to be locally administered at the discretion of the institutions. Such an arrangement, opined the MAC, "could relieve the central agency of the overwhelming task of administering small grants-in-aid." The Bowman Committee argued that funds should be available to accredited universities, colleges, and engineering schools "in a manner which will be virtually automatic." Once accepted in the plan, and as long as its bookkeepers knew the money was going for research, "[the institution] would expect to receive the grant as a regular annual appropriation." The Committee also felt the board must "be freed from the burden of investigating a large number of potential recipients [proposals] and judging the merits and defects of each." Each advisory group laid plans for provision of fellowships and grants, but these were to be smaller shares of the annual outlay.

One of the features of the Bowman Committee recommendations (that did not occur to the MAC) was the preference that universities obtain their money only on a *matching* basis. Was this to mean that the "Bowmanites," emboldened by the potential of the federal treasury, were regressing to the memories of an earlier pre-depression period? In the heyday of the Rockefeller Foundation, in 1910-1920, matching had been the primary mode of philanthropy. Abraham Flexner, who had a large role in assisting the Rockefeller philanthropies, had operated by a set of firm principles.[31] The first of these stipulated that "a large foundation should operate on a large plan, making its gifts by wholesale and not by retail." One of his corollary rules was that "a foundation can best justify its strategic position in our society by stimulating gifts from others, through the device of requiring that its gifts be matched." In recent times, the NSF has employed matching or *leverage* in some of its large award programs. Given the tightness of money in 1945, it would have been an inequitable way to start a new government program based on merit.

How to Cut a Pie

Bush proceeded to finish his reply to the President in the first week of June, 1945. His proposed NRF would have five divisions and be run by a board to whom the director would report. His divisions and their projected budgets (in $ millions) were:

	1st yr	5th yr
Medical Research	5	20
Natural Sciences	10	50
National Defense	10	20
Scientific Personnel and Education	7	29
Publications and Administration	1.5	3.5
Totals	33.5	122.5 [2]

Release of the Report

On June 14, Bush met with President Truman for about 15 minutes to gain the President's reaction to the report and obtain permission for its release. The President had read and liked the report.[17] The report was released to the press on July 19, 1945.[32,33] On the ABC radio network, the popular commentator Raymond Gram Swing was highly laudatory, and the press was generally favorable. *The New York Times*, however, ruffled feathers by an editorial position that the NRF seemed an inadequate instrument for overall government science planning. For this, publisher Arthur Hays Sulzberger received a rebuke from Conant,[34] and from his privileged view as a member of the Advisory Committee of the OSRD, James Phinney Baxter III advised the publisher that "Bush and Conant in the past five years have had experience vouchsafed to few of the difficulty of getting enough freedom inside the government structure to permit scientists to do their work effectively."[35]

The President was by now in Potsdam. His first meeting with Josef Stalin occurred shortly before he was informed of the successful first test of the atomic bomb at Alamagordo. This testimony to the potentially awesome power of government-funded S&T also must have been much on the mind of Vannevar Bush throughout this same period, for as OSRD director he was intimately involved with secret discussions, at the highest level, on how a successful experiment should be used to bring the war most quickly to an end.[36]

The description of the OSRD activities during the war, which was the first request in FDR's letter, had been of considerable importance to Vannevar Bush because he sought to counter a barrage of criticism directed at OSRD by Senator Harley Kilgore (D-W.Va.). Since 1942, Kilgore had attempted to pass legislation directed toward both tightening the government management of OSRD and broadened federal sponsorship of research, under conditions that Bush and many others steadfastly opposed.[17] By the time the Bush report was formally submitted to the President on July 25, a fresh draft of a new bill was released by Senator Warren Magnuson (D-Wash.); it filled Bush's prescription for the new science agency.[32]

Other Ambitions

Under a section entitled "Means to the End," Bush placed in his report stringent views on the competition for what was to be the National Research Foundation:

> There are within Government agencies many groups whose interests are primarily those of scientific research...These groups should remain as they are...they cannot be made the repository of new and large responsibilities for science which belong to the Government and which the Government should accept....Nowhere in the governmental structure receiving its funds from Congress is there an agency adapted to supplementing the support of basic research in universities.[2]

The National Institute of Health

In the early 1940s, there were over forty government research laboratories, and work in many of these was supported by OSRD contracts. Temporary laboratory buildings for this purpose had been erected on the 100-acre campus of the National Institute of Health in Bethesda, Maryland. The several hundred scientists in this facility were engaged in research in basic sciences, such as chemistry, physiology, nutrition, and microbiology. Scientists in other laboratories were concerned with the applied sciences, some related to "control" activities associated with the mandates of the United States Public Health Service. A large number of the scientists were PHS career officers, who worked alongside civilian scientists, a tradition maintained today. Many of the scientists had entered the PHS immediately upon receiving their advanced degrees. Some had acquired most or all of their scientific training in the PHS. Very few were trained for, or interested in, clinical medicine. Although a few were internationally recognized specialists in their disciplines, the majority of the scientific workers were on career paths less glamorous than those of the professors and academicians from the great universities and medical schools who made up the Bowman and MAC groups of advisors.

Nevertheless, the NIH scientists of the 1940s were no less jealous than the professors and academicians of the academic freedom accorded them at the NIH. They adhered to the proud and solid tradition of the Hygienic Laboratory that was opened in 1887 by the Marine Hospital Service, and which had been the predecessor of the NIH. Some of the older staff members had been among those opposed to the attempts of Senator Joseph Ransdell (D-La.) in the late 1920s to expand the Hygienic Laboratory.[37] Ransdell was pursuing a dream of creating a great medical research institution in which hundreds of scholars would work on the underlying basis of all the diseases of humankind. The scholars would be generously equipped, have access to a big library, and be surrounded by an army of research fellows and other trainees.[38]

Intramural opposition to Ransdell's ambition had existed within the scientific leadership of the Hygienic Laboratory. Arthur Stimson, head of the PHS Division of Scientific Research, was negatively inclined. Gene Dyer, a PHS-trained expert in rickettsia and acting director of the Hygienic Laboratory, thought that the expansion of a good laboratory should "... [proceed] in the light of a slow or deliberate growth rather than growth of a mushroom type."[37]

The Ransdell Act finally passed in 1930, but unfortunately at the very time when the nation was in the trough of the Great Depression. The legislative prize was reduced to a change of the name of the laboratory, a few hundred thousands of dollars for a new building, and the right to accept gifts. Authority for fellowships was granted, but with little in the way of funds to support them. Unseated at the next election, Ransdell dedicated several years to a fruitless pursuit of support, receiving a deaf ear from corporations and private givers alike.[36]

In the cadre of PHS officers at headquarters in the 1930s, however, there were some who were much less conservative than the majority, and they desired that considerably more attention be paid to the service's ability to fulfill its mandate to guard the public health. One group was particularly interested in the field operations. Another, smaller group was more desirous of enhancing basic and clinical science. Much later this difference of opinion would be expressed in the dominance of the bench scientists and bedside clinical researchers in Bethesda, with the more traditional public health field workers migrating to other posts. The latter group was exemplified by Joseph Mountin, an ebullient epidemiologist and inventive scientist who was considered by his peers as a "genius in the field."[39] Mountin became the "father" of what is today the Centers for Disease Control, an offshoot from NIH that moved to Atlanta in the early 1940s.

Thompson and Parran

Among those who dreamed of a great expansion of the scientific capabilities of the PHS in 1930, undoubtedly the most active was L. R. Thompson, who had just become chief scientist of the PHS. A kindred spirit was Thomas Parran, who had come to Washington in 1926 as head of the Division of Venereal Diseases. Both Thompson and Parran were visionaries, comfortable with the New Deal philosophy of federal activism that would come to Washington with the election of Franklin Delano Roosevelt in 1932. The names of

Thompson and Parran, along with that of Gene Dyer, are little-known to the present generation of medical scientists. Yet they constituted the trio of Public Health Officers destined to realize Ransdell's vision with creation of the modern NIH.

Thompson. Lewis Ryer Thompson, known universally as "Jimmie," was born in 1883.[40-42] His first job after graduating from Louisville Medical College was that of a quarantine officer in the Philippine Constabulary. After joining the PHS in 1910, his schooling in epidemiology, stream pollution, and disease control was highly practical and confined to field investigations. Thompson came to Washington in 1921 and was made the first chief of Industrial Hygiene Investigations in the PHS Division of Scientific Research. By the time he succeeded Stimson as chief of the latter division in 1930, he had already compensated for a lack of academic scientific training by a steadily growing mastery of the operations of the Congress and the federal bureaucracy.

Parran. The eventual achievements of Thomas Parran place him today in the first rank of all the surgeons general of the United States. He described himself as "coming from an impecunious, but proud background" in southern Maryland, and he never attended a formal school, receiving all of his education at home from an aunt-in-law before he entered St. John's College in Annapolis.[43] He graduated from Georgetown University Medical School in 1915. "Those days," he later recalled, "there were only three places in the country where a young physician could do good research, the Mayo Clinic, the Rockefeller Institute, and the Hygienic Laboratory. The Public Health Service was about the only place where one could do good research and receive some, what I call proper, pay for it."[42] Entering the PHS in 1917 after a year's internship in a private hospital in Washington, Parran obtained some microbiology training at the Hygienic Laboratory and soon after concentrated on field work in venereal diseases.

Parran and Thompson shared instinctively a commonality of interests in promoting the Public Health Service and were thus effective boosters of the fledgling NIH. They were willing to pull the tail of the establishment to further this ambition. An early act of collusion occurred immediately after passage of the Ransdell Act, when Thompson and Parran were among those dispatched to survey the proposed site of the new building at 25th and E Streets in Washington. The two returned with a dismal report, protesting that many times the available amount of space would be needed. Surgeon General Hugh Cumming and NIH Director George McCoy vigorously disagreed and were supported by their superior, Treasury Secretary Andrew Mellon, who felt that the several acres on the site would be enough for at least fifteen years.[44]

In 1930 Parran left Washington for Albany. New York's Governor Franklin Roosevelt had requested Surgeon General Cumming to detail an officer for the position of State Health Commissioner, and Parran was chosen. Parran was highly regarded in New York and proved to be an activist in awakening the state to the danger of denying that venereal disease was a serious health problem. On one occasion he said that he was abruptly taken off the air by CBS and replaced by piano music for uttering the word "syphilis" in a speech.[38] More important, as he worked among the hospitals and people of New York, Parran had experiences that reinforced a growing conviction that no time should be lost in starting a vigorous assault on the chronic diseases.

As the mortality among the young declined with increasing control of the infectious diseases, there was a reciprocal and sharply rising proportion of the burden of illness and disability in degenerative heart disease, cancer, and mental illness. Parran soon also realized that the campaign must begin with more research on these diseases, including clinical investigation, a view that much of the medical community felt was highly premature.

The friendship that evolved between Governor Roosevelt and Parran led in 1936 to Roosevelt's appointment of Parran to succeed Cumming as surgeon general. Long before he returned to Washington, Parran was kept busy drawing up plans for health reorganization in the administration of the newly elected President of the United States.

Jimmie's Capers

The Science Advisory Board. Thompson, described in a 1934 news clip as a "silver-haired official with golf-tanned arms...a cool official in a cool office on the third floor of the Public Health Service Building...,"[45] made the most of this office, which was conveniently located in the surgeon general's headquarters in the Treasury Department, the parent agency of the PHS from its inception as the Marine Hospital Service in 1798.

Thompson was in the halls of Congress before 1930 when Senator Ransdell needed a hand during the birth of the NIH.[46] The record abounds with instances when Thompson was able to make key plays in attempts to benefit PHS science.[47] For example, in 1934 Thompson was present when Compton's Science Advisory Board met with the Bureau of the Budget and Secretary of Agriculture Henry A. Wallace. Wallace, who had been brought up in a family business in developing corn hybrids, had more of a scientific bent than most persons who attain a cabinet post. He remarked that he favored "a very limited amount" of federal money as grants to universities for research. This statement caused Thompson considerable anxiety because he feared that the PHS might miss a possible opportunity to increase its own research funds in the wake of such a program. Wallace's subsequent suggestion to the President that the SAB membership include medical orientation allowed Thompson opportunity to engineer, through Secretary of the Treasury Henry A. Morganthau, two appointments. One of these was Parran, the other was Milton Rosenau, a Harvard epidemiologist and director of the Hygienic Laboratory between 1899 and 1909.

Thompson went further, again apparently inducing Secretary Morganthau to suggest to chairman Compton that the SAB detail a subcommittee to examine the research strength of the PHS.[47] Compton graciously agreed to do so and assigned the study to a Committee on Medical and Public Health Problems, consisting of the three physicians who had been newly appointed to the SAB, Parran, Rosenau, and NAS member Simon Flexner, nearing the end of his long and distinguished term as director of the Rockefeller Institute.[48] Thompson, unhappy with a copy of a draft report of the study he received from Rosenau, arranged to draft the report himself and sent it to Parran for approval of the other two members.[46]

The report of the committee on medicine and public health, released in March 1935, was all of twelve double-spaced pages and has to be regarded from today's perspective as a fairly naive "puff-piece."[49] The report began by listing some of the more outstanding discoveries of the PHS, which included important work on typhus and discovery of the cause of pellagra. Following this brief recital, however, the report abruptly ended in a recommendation that the funds for the scientific work of the PHS in the coming year be increased by $2 million. There was no plan or analysis of how this money was to be used, although it was a huge sum in those days, considering that the total budget of the PHS was $10 million, and most of it dedicated to maintaining the Marine Hospital Service. The final report of the SAB itself, which expired in December 1935, avoided mention of the health subcommittee's efforts.[48,50] The National Academy of Sciences wasted no time in replacing the SAB with a successor Government Relations & Science Advisory Group, a move that prevented the White House from again appointing an NAS committee, thereby overriding the academy charter established by President Woodrow Wilson.[51] The NAS just as promptly took steps to assure that non-NAS members Parran and Rosenau were not appointed to the SAB successor.[52]

NIH Moves to Bethesda. The PHS received no answer to its plea for increased funds through the SAB. Thompson also had no success in inducing the administration to take on one of the list of seventy "initiatives for new PHS research," which he released in August 1935.[53] Nevertheless, his connections and public relations skills paid off handsomely when, in the mid-1930s, another letter to the President came to his attention. This time it was an offer from the Luke Wilson family in Bethesda to donate some of their land to a worthy government purpose. Thompson arranged through Surgeon General Cumming to visit the Wilson family. At first, Thompson had in mind an animal farm for the NIH, still located in two adjacent buildings on the crowded site in Washington. As they grew to share Thompson's enthusiasm, however, the Wilsons eventually donated nearly 95 acres, the bulk of their estate, for relocation of the entire NIH from its Washington location.[39]

In 1937 Surgeon General Parran made the NIH his scientific division and appointed Thompson as director to succeed George McCoy, the nation's leading expert in leprosy, who had stubbornly resisted further expansion of NIH.[54] With Parran's White House connections, enough money was found to build two buildings. Parran turned the first spade in January 1938, and the cornerstone of Building One was laid in July. The trowel was given to Secretary Morganthau by the surgeon general.

The earliest NIH buildings bear the mark of Thompson's predilections in several ways. In 1936 Thompson had extended his attendance at an industrial hygiene meeting in Geneva to a three-month tour of state-supported research institutions in Europe and Scandinavia. His reports to the surgeon general were scholarly and analytically sound, as well as candid. He considered the Pasteur Institute to be a "benign dictatorship under Roux," the "salaries entirely inadequate," and the laboratories poorly supported.[55] One is compelled to believe, however, that Thompson had also carried back some favorable images of the world-famous institute, when one observes the mansard roofs and sizes of the first buildings constructed on the NIH campus. They too much resemble (in Georgian style) the architecture of the Pasteur and DuClaux buildings that face each other across the rue Dr. Roux in Paris. A further sign of Thompson's laboratory orientation is the official names he gave to the now-familiar first buildings on the campus: "Industrial Hygiene" for Building Two, "Public Health Methods" for Building Three, while Four and Five were the "Infectious Disease Buildings."

Cancer

The evidence that Congress was ready to use federal money to back medical research in public and private institutions—without benefit of the views of a Bowman Committee—was apparent before 1945.[56] Indeed, there had been vigorous congressional tugging on the bio-medical science culture warp since the 1920s. By 1944, there was enough evidence of increasing tension—in the moves to expand the

NIH—to give pause to those laboring to create a single agency for federal support of all science. If a relatively modest sector was being reserved for medical science, its subject matter was primed to expand explosively and could leave the fledgling NRF a shambles. The ultimate complicity of the medical academicians of the CMR and MAC in Bush's unitary theme can partly be attributed to Bush's strong personality. But possibly it was also related to a prevailing opinion that "public health research," as represented by the NIH, was mainly sanitary engineering, vaccination, and vital statistics, and not serious "fundamental" medical science. Whatever the cause, the NRF architects were deaf to the drums beating in the Congress.

Humanity's Most Deadly Scourge
"... a monster that is more insatiable than the guillotine, more destructive to life, health and happiness than the World War ... more irresistible than the mightiest army."
Senator Matthew Neeley, May 1928. [55]

In 1927 Senator Matthew Neeley (D-W.Va.) introduced a bill (S. 5589) to authorize a federal award for the cure to cancer. Rebuffed, a year later he proposed authorizing generous funding for the NAS to determine how the federal government should engage this enemy, which he described as "humanity's most deadly scourge" in a vivid polemic before the Congress.[55] At that time, Ransdell pointed out to Neeley that the PHS had been studying cancer since the early 1920s (including a cancer research unit at Harvard Medical School) and reminded him of the augmentation of such research already inherent in his drafts for upgrading the Hygienic Laboratory. The passage of Ransdell's bill in 1930 temporarily deflated the congressional pressure to mandate the support of a single disease.

When he became surgeon general, Parran was aware of both the concerns of Congress and the urging of a small but powerful group of public supporters. He therefore provided the Congress with the outlines of a national program for cancer control, which he believed must include stepped-up clinical research.[57] At about the same time, Dudley Jackson, a Texas internist, induced Congressman Maury Maverick (D-Tex.) to ask the NIH Director to help draft a bill for establishment of a National Cancer Institute (NCI), but no answer came from director George McCoy. Maverick persisted without such support and in April 1937 submitted a bill to create a cancer institute. It was just a few days after that a bill was submitted by Senator Homer Bone (D-Wash.), who had been assisted by Parran. A companion bill was submitted from the House by Congressman Magnuson.

At a joint hearing on the Cancer Act, Senator Bone remarked:

> I have received hundreds of letters urging passage of this bill. People all over the Nation are interested in any move to make real progress toward discovering the causes of this disease.[58]

His cosponsor, Senator Roy Copeland (D-N.Y.), added:

> The (bill is) introduced in the Senate jointly for myself and *for every member of the Senate*. In the 15 years during which I have been in the Senate, I have never known such a thing to happen before.[57]

On July 27, 1937, the House approved the Senate's joint National Cancer Act, and President Roosevelt made it law on August 5.[59] The new institute was fitted with a National Advisory Cancer Council (NACC), similar to the National Advisory Health Council (NAHC) established for the NIH in 1930. The NACC was to approve extramural grants made for cancer research. This key provision of the National Cancer Act did not receive adequate funding until about 1945.

The cancer movement thus was now established within the NIH. The restless anxiety of its fervent supporters would reappear again and again in the future, creating tension with the attempts of the NIH leadership to maintain an integrated program of research on human biology and disease. Such separation early manifested itself in a movement to have a hospital for cancer alone in Bethesda. More serious was the barely averted schismatic movement in the early 1970s, arising from efforts to increase cancer funding.[60]

On the other hand, parochial stimulation of more support for cancer frequently has proved to be a boon for the whole of biomedical research, because of the "Venetian structure of NIH" created by the early grants program officers. This means that on the surface each of the major disease categories is visible; beneath, the support is largely miscible, allowing growth of all the biomedical disciplines.[61] By 1944 "The Most Deadly Scourge" had become the strongest thread in the medical science culture warp.

Public Law 78-410.

When the U.S. entered World War II, the Public Health Service had to turn its attention to greatly expanded responsibilities, but planning for increasing capacity was not entirely neglected. In 1942 Dyer succeeded Thompson as NIH director and assumed his seat on the CMR. Though ailing, Thompson became in charge of legislative matters and for several years concentrated on assisting Congressman Alfred Lee Bulwinkle (D-N.C.), who was chairman of a subcommittee of the House Interstate and Foreign Commerce Committee that was seeking to straighten out the "messy structure" of public health laws. Hearings, beginning July 1, 1944, on a Public Health Service Act featured a long appearance by Parran and a good deal of careful chairmanship by Bulwinkle to reassure some conservative Republican members that several new authorities proposed for the surgeon general were not novel but derived from existing law.[62] In this way, the National Cancer Act became particularly helpful because Congressman Bulwinkle could point out that if the law allowed NCI to award extramural research grants, of course this authority should also be given to the NIH. In the language of the new legislation, the NCI—at Parran's insistence—was bound firmly into the family, as a ninth division of the NIH.

Section 301 in this act gave the PHS, through the surgeon general, almost unlimited authority to perform and support extramural biomedical research. The new powers derived from what became Public Law 78-410 had yet to be tested before the President's November 1944 letter initiated the actions of Vannevar Bush.

"(d) Make grants-in-aid to universities...and other public or private institutions, and to individuals for such research projects as are recommended by the NAHC or NACC."
From Section 301, Public Law 78-410 (1944)

The surgeon general had also not neglected other plans for peacetime expansion. Two weeks before the President's letter to Bush, Parran issued a "Ten Year Postwar

Program" for the PHS. It was cast in the frame of the activist New Deal adherent that he was. The plan advocated that "...there be available to everyone all medical and health services," public funds for implementation of a national medical care program, and, inter alia, public support of research. Plans for $23 million in new construction were detailed for the first postwar year. The top priority was allotted to a 500-bed hospital on the NIH campus.[63]

Letter to A. N. Richards. When the intent to demobilize the OSRD was taken up in the August 1944 meetings of the CMR, Gene Dyer, emboldened with the brand-new strength of P.L. 78-410, had expressed the view that the Public Health Service could take over contracts appropriate to its functions. A week later, with the concurrence of the surgeon general, he wrote a letter to Richards,[64] pointing out in detail the new authorities now held by the surgeon general and committing the PHS to assume the financial and scientific responsibilities of the (expiring) CMR. Dyer offered to appoint the personnel from DMS now advising the CMR to an advisory committee created for the National Advisory Health Council.

The letter was annexed to the minutes of the next CMR meeting, and referred to by Bush in a letter to Richards on September 18.[65] The PHS position was supported by some members of the CMR staff. James Moore, a top staff executive, wrote Bush's executive officer that if OSRD was to go, the CMR should be continued by a governmental body, "alternatively the NAS+NRC [sic] or the USPHS." Moore was fully aware of the new PHS authorities but noted that PHS policies would have to be "retooled," especially the relationships between the PHS research and that supported by extramural grants.[66] Perhaps because Bush was now busy with preparing a new agency, the CMR—and the PHS—waited for months for some signal of further demobilization. By May 1945, the DMS division chiefs decided to recommend that all contracts be transferred to other agencies at the end of the year. In June, Bush asked the CMR to stay fluid but by August 24 he sent Richards a set of principles by which the contracts should be organized for possible demobilization. These guidelines specified that military projects should be transferred to the military. Nonmilitary projects should be divided into one of three groups: (1) projects for private sponsorship by groups willing to be responsible for them; (2) projects properly within the scope of the PHS and which the PHS is willing to undertake; these would carry the funds budgeted for their continuance during the current fiscal year; and (3) projects which could best be furthered under the auspices of a federal agency will be continued with the expectation that such a federal agency will be created by the Congress.[64] Vannevar Bush's precise deadline for release had passed into the hands of Congress.

LEGISLATIVE CONFLICT

Different Concepts of an NRF

Four days after Senator Magnuson and others had introduced S.1285 to establish in law the Bush blueprint for the NRF, Sen. Harley Kilgore (D-W.Va.) and several colleagues introduced S.1297, a bill with a different model. This bill reflected what some considered a more populist or "socialist" view of government support of science, ideas that Kilgore had been revising and refining since 1942 in a legislative attempt to have the government more actively control the OSRD.[67] Kilgore's scheme called for a strong director, government retention of patents on discoveries arising from government-supported work, a distribution of 25 percent of the funds to the states for their tax-supported and land grant schools, not less than 15 percent of the total for medical research, and inclusion of the social sciences.[68] Most of this was anathema to Bush, but President Truman let it be known in a public statement that he favored the inclusion of the social sciences and certain other aspects of the Kilgore bill. Bush wrote a long letter to President Truman discussing the two bills and his opposition to Kilgore's version. He also complained to the President that, although he was nominally the science advisor, he had not been consulted by Truman before his recent message to Congress on science and research. The President and Bush had a conference on these differences,[69] but, as Bush complained later, he and the President never had a comfortable relationship.[9]

The Scientists Mobilize. Overwhelmingly in favor of the Magnuson version, the scientists and institutional leaders organized to support it. Many of them testified in Congress, wrote the President, and signed petitions to back Bush.[70]

In November, as the hearings bogged down, a Committee Supporting the Bush Report was founded by Isaiah Bowman. Its members tended to be the scientific elite including the MAC. However, the scientists were not of one mind as to tactics. Within a short time, another committee organized by Harold Urey and Harlow Shapley and supported by Einstein, Fermi, and Oppenheimer backed a compromise bill.[17] The Bowman committee sent a letter to the President endorsed by its adherents. By December 1945, the signatories numbered 1377 academicians. More than half (727) of these were deans, department heads, professors, and staff of medical schools; others were biologists (295), chemists (150), and physicists (104). This letter opposed the inclusion of the social sciences as well as the appointment by the President of a strong director; the letters also insisted that the governing authority should rest with the board.[69]

One of the many who testified in Congress for the Magnuson bill was Milislav Demerec, director of both the Biological Laboratory and the Carnegie Department of Genetics at Cold Spring Harbor:

> Moreover, it has been found in practice that placing fundamental research under the control of agencies that anticipate practical applications seriously limits and restrains the freedom of thought essential for basic advances.[71]

These sentiments could not have gone unnoticed in Bethesda. There was no doubt, however, that many basic scientists were alarmed that a section of the Magnuson bill included a Section 5, that read:

> (1) A Division of Medical Research: Programs relating to research in the biological sciences, including medicine and related sciences.

To soothe the basic scientists' fears, Homer Smith wrote a letter on behalf of the Medical Advisory Committee pointing out that the MAC "had never considered the biological sciences within its scope."[72] After the hearings, a compromise bill (S.1850) was approved by both sides. It appeared that the OSRD was to be transferred to a National Science Foundation. The compromise bill passed the Senate, but the House adjourned while the bill was still before a committee.[73]

Contracts Released

As the Congress deliberated through August, time seemed to be running out. The division chiefs pushed for transfer of the contracts lest they all expire before a new agency was created. They would use the classification that Bush had ordered. In the first week of September 1945, Dyer received notice from A. N. Richards:

> In order that disposition of active CMR contracts can be arranged, it is desirable that a meeting of the CMR Division Chiefs and yourself or your authorized representative be held...at the NAS on September 5.[74]

The minutes of the next CMR meeting on September 6 are anticlimactic.[75] There is attached without comment an annex reading:

> 2. Disposition of our Contracts. DIV I Medicine Recommended for Transfer to US PHS. Medicine, (39 contracts) for $662,000; blood studies, (5) for $65,000; chemistry, (2) for $12,000.

The total of all CMR contracts outstanding came to $2,127,000, about two-thirds of which were marked as reserved for "to new foundation," or "to be kept by CMR." The minutes were bare of details and suggested none of the high drama as related by A. Baird Hastings. This charter member of the CMR delighted in describing the final moments thus: "As Richards offered up each contract, only Gene Dyer made a bid, and afterwards he calmly walked home with the bundle."[76]

THE BATON IS PASSED

Ambivalence

It is obvious that the transfer of the CMR contracts to the NIH on September 6 were not perceived, either by the scientists in general or the biomedical community in particular, as the beginning of the Millennium. Presumably most still believed that the Bush model would emerge within the next Congress. None could foresee that during 1946 the legislators would have to concentrate on the creation of a new government keeper to husband the mixed blessing of atomic fission. The establishment of the Atomic Energy Agency also put in place an unforeseen new mission agency for science. A year later, President Truman, determined to have an NSF director responsible to him and not to a board, vetoed the NSF legislation. The accouchement of NSF was beset with unbearably prolonged labor pains.

The two major science advisory councils responsible to the NIH were equally nonplussed by the opportunity that had been thrust upon their agency and the challenge of shaping future biomedical research. On September 29, nearly a month after the CMR contracts had been moved, a joint meeting of the National Advisory Health Council and the National Advisory Cancer Council was convened. The agenda featured a debate over the new Division of Medical Sciences of the NRF in the plan proposed by Vannevar Bush. Dr. Parran informed the council members of the transfer of CMR grants to NIH that had very recently taken place. In a seemingly routine performance of its statutory duties, the NAHC reviewed and approved the renewal of the contracts Dyer had brought home as well as the seeking of a supplemental appropriation of about $900,000 that would be necessary to meet this obligation.

However, when the question was considered of whether the Public Health Service should take on the responsibility for grants in medical research, the majority of the members were against the idea on the grounds that the responsibilities for such grants were: (a) too great an added burden for the PHS, and (b) more appropriately belonged to the agency administering similar programs in other scientific fields, including the basic sciences related to medical science. A subcommittee consisted of the leading basic scientist on each council: Andrew Ivy, the famed physiologist from Chicago, and the biochemist William C. Rose, a pioneer in essential amino acids at the University of Illinois. The two were appointed to draw up a resolution. The drafters produced a statement that both advisory councils thought the PHS should retain its independence and expand its *own* [emphasis mine] research. The resolution passed.[77]

Appropriations Test. Gene Dyer, the son of a clergyman, went to Kenyon College and the University of Texas Medical School. He had most of his years in the PHS in the Hygienic Laboratory and there had acquired a national reputation as an expert on epidemic typhus. , Old-timers at NIH describe him as an introspective man, reserved, polite, and the "quintessential bench scientist." Most seemed quite unaware of the tiger poised behind this dignified facade. Guided by Parran, Dyer was unperturbed by the criticism and ambivalence of both the NIH advisory councils and the greater biomedical community. He immediately turned to "get funds for them" (the contracts) and "see to it that the program was put into the hands of scientists and kept there honestly."[78]

The OSRD had convinced the Bureau of the Budget that money should be transferred to the Public Health Service to cover a one-year renewal of the contracts it had taken home. The House appropriations subcommittee, however, objected to this tactic, and insisted upon hearing a proposal for a supplemental appropriation to the PHS Fiscal '47 budget that had previously been approved. On April 10, 1946 Dyer appeared before Congressman Albert L. Engel (R.-Mich.), the ranking minority member of the appropriations subcommittee responsible for the Federal Security Agency, which in 1939 had become the location of the PHS. Engel, who had been intimately involved in the funding of the work on the atom bomb and other high technology projects through service on another appropriations subcommittee, was thoroughly familiar with the OSRD. Thus the following colloquy between the two men, here presented in its entirety, can be passed off as merely a good example of the genre of congressional theater known as "making a record." To those, however, who like to savor the historical symbolism of American biomedical science passing from a shallow and uncertain bay into deep and unlimited waters, the following has a Homeric quality:

Mr. Engel: What was the supplemental of $1,178,000 for in FY '46?

Dr. Dyer: $817,000 of that was a supplemental appropriation for research grants.

Mr. Engel: Grants-in-aid to the States?

Dr. Dyer:	Not grants-in-aid to the States, but . . . for research work. We took over contracts for OSRD at their request.
Mr. Engel:	What is the OSRD?
Dr. Dyer:	The Office of Scientific Research and Development. That was the office which handled the atomic bomb research, medical research and other research.
Mr. Engel:	What was the date you took over this work?
Dr. Dyer:	On the 1st of January (1946).[79]

Philosophical Adaptations

The surgeon general established a Division of Research Grants in 1946. Dyer chose C. J. Van Slyke, a former field worker in venereal disease control, to take responsibility for the grants. One of the reasons for Dyer's choice was that Van Slyke, a gruff and capable man, was free because he was just recovering from a myocardial infarction and Dyer thought the job would not take too much of his day. Van Slyke, in turn, chose Ernest Allen and a few other helpers. They wasted no time in assembling study sections. By mid-1946 10 study sections were established and more added rapidly to make 21 by the end of the year. The sections covered *basic science disciplines* such as pharmacology and bacteriology; *diseases*, like syphilis and malaria; and *systems,* such as cardiovascular, which included both basic science and clinical medicine.

From the first day, the study section membership was siphoned from elite pools, including many advisers from the DMS committees that had assisted the CMR. Of the 75 medical scientist members of the NAS in 1946, 12 were members of the first study sections.[80,81] James A. Shannon, then at the Squibb Institute, was the chairman of the malaria study section, and Johns Hopkins' E. Cowles Andrus chaired the cardiology section. These were roles they had played for the CMR. About 1000 proposals were received the first year, and the amount awarded came to $5.5 million.

Among the dozen or so study fields in the first year, syphilis was the leader in dollar volume of grants, followed by cardiology and physiology. The leading states in terms of number of grantees were, in descending order, New York, Massachusetts, Illinois, Pennsylvania, and California.[80]

The ascent of the annual NIH obligations for extramural research grants was swift. The approximately $4 million in fiscal year 1947 rose to $15.6 million in fiscal year 1950, to $36.6 million in 1955, and by 1960 was $203 million. This last figure represented two-thirds of all NIH obligations in 1960 ($338 million).[82]

By 1948 officials from the Bureau of the Budget and the Federal Security Agency were urging NIH to resist cloning of the institute model for any more diseases.[83] A Mental Health Institute had already been authorized, with pressure on the Congress from professionals and laymen.[84] A single anecdote may suffice to illustrate the ferment of the late forties. Leonard Scheele, who served as director of the Cancer Institute from July 1947 until he was appointed surgeon general in April 1948, later recalled his participation in the following notes as recorded by his interviewer:

> Mary Lasker [asked] 'Len, why shouldn't there be a Heart Institute?' Len wrote the bill [slightly revising the National Cancer Act]... Dyer gave OK...,Parran blessing... Lasker got bill to [Senator] Styles Bridges...on President's desk 'for weeks'.[85]

There were many others in addition to Mrs. Lasker who contributed to the accelerated pluralization of the NIH. This was a period of giddy growth that saw both heart and dental institutes arrive in 1948. Before long, many citizen activists urged a willing Congress to eventually extend the attack on all diseases, as had been Ransdell's dream. These expansive adjustments of the culture warp are themes for other essays and beyond the scope of this story.

Project or Institutional Grants. Almost reflexly, Van Slyke and his team had adopted the project grant as the principal basis for the extramural program. There is very little evidence that the Congress initially planned this approach, although it has been pointed out by Donald Price, who was on the scene, that Congress recognized it would have a difficult time making awards to institutions with their different public and private, sometimes religious origins. It was easier to let the peer review process make the choices with delegation of the final responsibility to the advisory councils that also had public representatives.[86]

It is often pointed out that project grant had become the preferred mechanism of support by the largest philanthropic organizations before the war, after the bulk grant to institutions had become both boring and no longer financially feasible. One of the impresarios of such support for small groups of gifted investigators was the Rockefeller Foundation's Warren Weaver, a member of the Bowman Committee.[87] He and his fellow foundation administrators had promulgated a "best science" tradition that has dominated funding of science for this century. The probable reason for the NIH project grant choice was that NIH wanted to take over where the OSRD had left off, to choose individuals or small groups of investigators for individual awards. In Van Slyke's 1946 description of the intent of the NIH extramural program, he described it as resting "on the integrity and independence of research workers, and their freedom from control, regimentation and outside interference."[88] Dyer later echoed these sentiments: "...emphasis is placed not on the goal, but upon the scientist pursuing interests as distinct from bureaucratic control over those interests."[89] Doubtless they firmly believed these concepts, but they also were aware that the scientific community was scrutinizing them carefully for any of the dread signs of the predicted inability of a government mission agency to run a grants program adhering strictly to the already established "best science" tradition.

Roger L. Geiger viewed this community reaction as a natural one. The Depression had ended the dependence of the university basic research on philanthropic sources; the superimposition of any federal funding agency on the existing system would be intolerable if it failed to allow the scientists and their institutions "to retain freedom of scientific research, peer control and the autonomy of the universities."[90] To be sure, the 'autonomy' of the universities was initially altered greatly by the NIH granting practices. A peer-regulated decision process operating distal to the universities was put in place to determine which of their faculty members would be supported to do research work. The institutions would not make that decision at home.

At first, neither the early NIH administrators, who were busy establishing their credibility as effective heirs of the OSRD, nor the outside community, which was busy monitoring the NIH performance, were paying proper mind to the future. It seemed likely that in the long run the strictly categorical, highly targeted project grants appropriate for the OSRD would not give the ideal coverage of science that could be obtained on broader long-term support for the best minds. This may have justifiably bothered some supporters of broad institutional support even though the NIH approach pleased the rank and file of scientists. With the exception of the needs of fledgling scientists and others caught between grants, most scientists today probably believe that the university is not in the best position to allocate support to its faculty investigators strictly on merit. However, in 1955 there was a short-lived attempt to resurrect the arguments for institutional-based funding held by the Bowman Committee and the MAC.

Brief Revolt. Soon after she took over as overseer of the Public Health Service in 1953, Secretary Oveta Culp Hobby of the Department of Health, Education, and Welfare ordered an outside study of the NIH research programs. In accord with its recent mandate,[91] the National Science Foundation, which had at last been created in 1950, was given responsibility for the study. The agency convened a special committee for this purpose consisting of university scientists under the chairmanship of C. N. H. Long, dean of Yale's medical school. The committee recommended that the NIH extramural grant program be severed from the intramural program. Furthermore, the Long committee indicated that the desired mode of research support was through "unrestricted institutional grants" to the school. However, events had overtaken this simpler vision, vintage 1945.

James A. Shannon, then the NIH director, thundered against such a fission of NIH. A new HEW Secretary, Marion Folsom, appointed his own investigating committee, headed by Dr. Stanhope Bayne-Jones, who had been another Yale dean. Senator Lister Hill (D-Ala.), now in the chair of both the Senate authorizing and appropriations subcommittees with jurisdiction over NIH, asked an educator, Dr. Boisfeuillet Jones, to conduct his own study for the

Congress. Both reviews disagreed strongly with the NSF study committee. The committee report, never officially published, lies in the archives.[92]

Basic v. Applied Research. In 1947 nearly everyone in the academic community appeared to share a canonical belief that, as Bush implied in his report (and Demerec and others had echoed in testimony and private sentiments), an agency doing applied research could not be entrusted with handling basic research. In fact, one of Bush's five principles for operation of the new agency was that it was not to operate any laboratories of its own.[2] As Homer Smith's disclaimer[72] revealed, the members of the MAC in 1945 seemed astonishingly unaware of the concept that between the most fundamental biology and clinical research there stretches an uninterrupted continuum. From ancient times, medicine has always been one of the best tutors of biology. Yet the former cannot survive without constant refreshment from the deeper wells of fundamental discovery. The several founders of the modern NIH left little written evidence that they understood completely how close was the interrelationship, but in their actions they helped anneal forever the linkage between basic and applied biomedical research.

The story of how they built the largest laboratory in the world for unequivocal demonstration of this linkage is too long to tell here. It is important to note, however, that it was during the same appropriations hearings in which Dyer had carried the OSRD contracts over the great divide, that he and Parran also pledged to return the following year to obtain a commitment to build the NIH Clinical Center. The opportunity to do so had been opened by the insertion of another clause into Section 301 of P.L. 78-410 that allowed patients to be admitted for purposes of research only.

" **(f) For purposes of study, admit and treat...persons not otherwise eligible. . . "**
Section 301, Public Law 78-410

In the planning for the hospital, Parran and Dyer instinctively had to defend what is today recognized as a major principle of biomedical research, i.e., that maintaining the unity of biomedical and behavioral research in the immediate environment of clinical studies is the most effective way to understand disease. Repeatedly these two pioneers had to intervene to convince cancer and mental health researchers that one hospital was better than three.

Ground was broken in 1948 for an enormous new focus of the intramural program—a house that was described by one of its principal architects, Jack Masur, as containing "500 beds wrapped in a thousand laboratories." Construction would cost more than twice the sum expended by the CMR during the entire duration of the war. It frightened many of the NIH scientists at the time, just as Ransdell's plan had done decades before. Arthur Kornberg was one of those who left and provided a reflection on why in a recent book:

> The decision to go...turned out to be [two] errors in judgement. First I believed that the advent of the Clinical Center and the disease-oriented institutes would stifle basic research at NIH...[93]

Many in the academic community were angered by the building of so colossal a facility. Their representatives on the MAC had already expressed their opinion to Bush, which he had included in his report.

> "...we should set out to improve the research staffs and facilities of the present medical schools before we undertake the establishment of new institutions."

Now that the full support of the government had swung to biomedical research, this reading of the situation by the medical elect was too narrow.

When the Clinical Center opened in 1953, clinical investigation in America had indeed moved a great distance from the turn of the century. In 1910, a time when philanthropy provided what government would not, the Hospital of the Rockefeller Institute was opened as a unique model for the world.[94] The timing was right. Clinical research laboratories appeared in teaching hospitals in the Northeast: Philadelphia (1885), Baltimore (1907), New York City (1910-20), Boston (1922-25), and had become incubators for clinical researchers.[27] By 1950 one could say that the gap between the bedside and the laboratory was nearly closed. The difference ultimately provided in Bethesda was an interface between basic science and clinical research of such overwhelming density that the conversion of clinical investigation from an avocation to a full-time profession was greatly accelerated.[95] The virtue of fostering fundamental research in the vicinity of clinical medicine soon became a necessity for the advances against chronic diseases that had finally begun. The return of increasing numbers of scientists from the Clinical Center to the medical schools helped scatter across the nation, and to many parts of the world, the paradigm of how best to focus the knowledge available on human diseases.

Vannevar Bush deserves the high esteem that history has accorded him for singular achievements in times when the culture of American scientific endeavor and the associated institutions were changing from a predominately private mode to a public one. Those who assisted Bush in this transition made important contributions to laying out the defense of the scientific method and of the limits of its adjustment to the forces that support it. In doing so they positively influenced the transition to a partnership with the state and passed on passionate instruction on principles that endure today. Credit for the effective translation of these principles is owed to a small group of PHS officers, like Thompson,[96] Parran,[97] Dyer, and Van Slyke, who had the vision, character, and sense of public duty necessary to make the system work.

The culture warp too endures. Inseparable from the support and the substance of the weaving of knowledge, it will forever be a part of scientific inquiry. The complex network of forces involved in the public support and associated governance of biomedical science have together achieved a remarkable result in America.

Nevertheless, as the tapestry thickens and becomes more intricate, so does the warp. Capricious adjustments in the loom have become common. Too often, unthinking or selfish moves are made that increase the tension and the danger of snags that may seriously threaten the integrity and completeness of the fabric of knowledge. Because the loom belongs to civilization, anyone who attempts to change the function to suit his own design can put at risk all the generations yet to come.

Notes

1. Report of the Carnegie Commission on Science, Technology and Government. *Enabling the future: Linking science and technology to societal goals*. Washington, DC: Carnegie Commission; 1992.
2. Bush V. *Science, the Endless Frontier, A Report to the President on a Program for Postwar Scientific Research*. Washington, DC: National Science Foundation; 1960.
3. Preparation of this essay has included inspection of evidence in the National Archives, the Archives of the National Academy of Sciences, and the History of Medicine Division at the National Library of Medicine (NLMHMD) along a trail blazed by Donald Swain[4] and later extended by Daniel Fox,[5] and Stephen Strickland.[6] The search has included the NIH Central Files (NIHCF).
4. Swain DC. The Rise of a Research Empire: NIH, 1930-1950. *Science*. 1962;138:1233-1237.
5. Fox DM. Politics of the NIH Extramural Program, 1937-1950. *J. of History of Medicine and Applied Science*. 1987;42:447-466.
6. Strickland SP. *The Story of the NIH Grants Program*. New York, NY: University Press of America;1989.
7. Baxter III JP. *Scientists Against Time*. Boston, MA:Little Brown;1946.
8. Irvine S. *Organizing Scientific Research for War*. Boston, MA:Little Brown;1948.
9. Bush V. *Pieces of the Action*. New York, NY:Morrow;1970.
10. Harvey AM. *The Association of American Physicians 1886-1986*. Baltimore, MD:Waverly Press;1986.
11. Watson EL. *Houses for Science: A pictorial history of Cold Spring Harbor Laboratory*. Cold Spring Harbor, NY:Cold Spring Harbor Laboratory Press;1991.
12. National Archives RG 227 OSRD, Records of the OSRD, Records of the CMR; Minutes, Box 8, 8\3\44 to 12\21\44, Folders Aug 3, 1944 and Aug 17, 1944.
13. Roosevelt FD. Letter to Vannevar Bush. *JAMA*. 1944;126:904.
14. Gunther J. *Taken at the Flood*. New York, NY:Harper Brothers;1960.
15. Rosenman, S. Letter to Calvin B. Baldwin, Jr., April 5, 1961.
16. Rosenberg AM. Letter to Calvin B. Baldwin, Jr. April 27, 1961.
17. *England JM. A patron for pure science: the National Science Foundation's formative years, 1945-57*. Washington, DC:National Science Foundation;1982.
18. Cochrane RC. *The National Academy of Sciences: The First Hundred Years 1863-1963*. Washington, DC: National Academy of Sciences; 1978.
19. Archives of the National Academy of Sciences. Bowman Committee report on federal aid to research activities, 1944-45. Folder Executive Office for Emergency Management: OSRD;1944-45.
20. National Archives RG 227. OSRD, Office Chm NDRC and Dir. OSRD, corr. re Report to President 1941-46 Box 2 "Science the Endless Frontier." Folder General: Committee #2. Letter Vannevar Bush to A.N. Richards, November 18, 1944.
21. National Archives RG 227 OSRD, Records of the OSRD, Records of the CMR Minutes Box 8 8-3-44 to 12\21\44. Minutes of December 1, 1944.
22. Ibid. Box 8 CMR. Letter from Vannevar Bush to Walter W. Palmer, December 7, 1944; letter from Vannevar Bush to Homer W. Smith, December 20, 1944.
23. National Archives RG 227 OSRD, Records of the OSRD, Records of the CMR, Box 9 CMR Minutes of Jan. 18, 1945. Letter Vannevar Bush to A.N. Richards.
24. Archives of the National Academy of Sciences. Folder Executive Office for Emergency Mgt. OSRD 1944-45. Letter Frank Jewett to Vannevar Bush, June 6, 1945.
25. National Archives RG 227 OSRD, Office Chm NDRC and Dir. OSRD, corr. re Reports to President Box 1 "Science the Endless Frontier." Folder "General" 1\11\45 to 4\15\45.
26. Ibid. Letter Homer Smith to Vannevar Bush, March 6, 1945.
27. Medical Research Council Jubilee 1913-1963. *Brit Med J*. Nov 23, 1963.
28. Kohler RE. *From Medicinal Chemistry to Biochemistry*. Cambridge: Cambridge University Press; 1982.
29. National Archives RG 227 OSRD, Office Chm NDRC and Dir. OSRD, corr. re Reports to Bush, President Box 2 "Science the Endless Frontier." Folder "General" Reports. Memorandum "L.F.K." May 12, 1945.
30. National Archives RG 227 OSRD, Office Chm NDRC and Dir. OSRD, corr. re Reports to

President 1941-46. Box 1 Folder "Misc. 4\15\45 to 5\16\45.", Letter W.W. Palmer to V. Bush, April 25, 1945.

31. Flexner A. *An Autobiography*. New York, NY:Simon and Schuster; 1960.

32. Archives of The National Academy of Sciences. OSRD Release, July 19, 1945. Folder Executive Office for Emergency Management: OSRD: 1944-45.

33. National Archives RG 227 OSRD, Office Chm NDRC and Dir. OSRD, corr. re Reports to President 1941-46. Box 1 "Science the Endless Frontier." Folder "General, Pres. letter 11\17\44."

34. Ibid. Letter J.B. Conant to A.H. Sulzberger, August 14, 1945.

35. Ibid. Letter J.P. Baxter III to A.H. Sulzberger, August 20, 1945.

36. McCullough D. *Truman*. New York, NY: Simon and Schuster; 1992.

37. Harden VA. *Inventing the NIH: Federal Biomedical Research Policy, 1887-1937*. Baltimore, MD: Johns Hopkins University Press;1986.

38. NLMHMD. Box nho. Unpublished manuscript by Wyndam Miles on the establishment of the National Institutes of Health. p 16.

39. Armstrong BF. *A Profile of the United States Public Health Service, 1798-1948*. Washington, DC: DHEW Publication No. 73-369; 1973.

40. National Archives. RG 443. Records of L.R. Thompson, National Institute of Health 30-48. Box 197, Folder "personal history/LR Thompson."

41. National Archives RG 443. General Records, National Institute of Health 1930-48. Box 4 Folder "Cornerstone, Bethesda, June 30, 1938." NLMHMD. Box nho, Statement by Jimmie Thompson, Director of NIH, Placed in cornerstone of Building One, May 26, 1938.

42. Obituary, Lewis Ryer Thompson. *JAMA*. 1955;157:60 .

43. NLMHMD, MS C 203, Box P-V Interview with Thomas Parran, Rosen, George. Transcripts of Oral History Project.

44. Harden V. *Inventing the NIH:Federal Biomedical Research Policy, 1887-1937*.

45. National Archives. RG 443. Records of L.R. Thompson, National Institute of Health 30-48. Box 197, Folder "Personal History/Dr. Thompson." Clipping from United States News, August 13, 1934.

46. National Archives RG 443. Records of L.R.Thompson. National Institute of Health 30-48. Box 197, Folder "Discussion of S. 1171."

47. National Archives RG 443, Public Health Service Records 1930-48. Box 189. Folders "Science Advisory Board, corr. with Parran," and "Corr. with Rosenau."

48. Archives of the National Academy of Sciences. Ex.B. Science Advisory Board, Committee on Medicine and Public Health. Letter from Henry Morganthau, Jr., to Karl T. Compton, November 14, 1934. Letter from Karl T. Compton to Secretary Morganthau, November 27, 1934.

49. Archives of the National Academy of Sciences, Science Advisory Board, Committee on Medicine and Public Health. Report. March 1, 1935.

50. National Archives RG 443 General Records NIH 1930-48. Box 55 Folder "SAB."

51. Cochrane (17) provides details on the Science Advisory Board and Swain (4) sketches the PHS involvement. Thompson's role is revealed in (46) and (49).

52. Archives of the National Academy of Sciences. Executive Board SAB, Committee on Medicine and Public Health. Letter from Albert Barrows to Karl T. Compton, January 10, 1936.

53. Archives of the National Academy of Sciences. News release from Public Health Service, August 22, 1935. Executive Board Science Advisory Board, Committee on Medicine and Public Health.

54. Armstrong (38) and Harden (36) describe reactions of the old guard to Thompson's persistent attempts to "change the NIH into a major medical machine to fight chronic diseases." Director McCoy observed to his deputy Dyer that "We've got two buildings and NIH needs no more space than that."

55. National Archives RG 443 Records of L.R. Thompson National Institute of Health 30-48. Box 197 Folder "Dr.Thompson's European Reports."

56. Yaremchuk W. (The Cancer War: The Movement to Establish the National Cancer Institute, 1927-1937. Ph.D. diss., New York University, 1977.) has assembled the rhetoric and actions of this emotional period.

57. National Archives RG 443 General Records, NIH 1930-48 Box 6 Folder "Cancer." Carl

Voegtlin, NIH cancer researcher in a letter to SG Cumming, in 1929 strongly disagrees with the position of Dr. James Ewing, of New York's Memorial Hospital that more fundamental research must precede clinical research in cancer. Letter Surgeon General Parran to Senator Homer Bone, March 19,1937.

58. Joint hearings before a Subcommittee on Cancer Research of the Committee on Commerce, and Subcommittee on Cancer Research of the Committee on Interstate and Foreign Commerce, U.S. Senate; 5th Congress, 1st Session. July 8, 1937; Washington, DC.

59. Jimmie Thompson confided in his message left in the cornerstone of Bldg 1(40) that, under the direction of the Surgeon General, he wrote the Cancer bill, took care of "the arrangements for the hearings, which Senator Copeland kindly left in my hands," and wrote as well the House report on it. Ironically, Mr. Luke Wilson had died of cancer in June 1937. The family granted another ten acres for construction of a building for the cancer institute, on the NIH grounds.

60. Rettig RA. *Cancer Crusade: National Cancer Act of 1971*. Princeton, NJ: Princeton Univ. Press; 1977.

61. Fredrickson, DS. "Venice" is not sinking (the water is rising): Some views on biomedical research. *JAMA*. 1982;247:3072.

62. NLMHMD Box nho, Folder 1944-45 legislation. House Committee on Interstate and Foreign Commerce; Senate Committee on Labor and Education, Summary of P.L. 78-410, based on HR 4624 (Bulwinkle) July 1, 1944; Washington, DC.

63. NLMHMD C 204 Parran, Thomas, M.D. Proposed Ten-Year Postwar Program of the United States Public Health Service, November 1, 1944; Washington, DC.

64. National Archives RG 227 OSRD, Records of the CMR, Minutes Boxes 8 and 9 Folders Aug 17 minutes and "Aug 31, 1944. Letter from Rolla Dyer to A.N. Richards, August 29, 1944.

65. Stewart I. p 314-316.

66. National Archives RG 227 OSRD, Office Chm NDRC and Dir. OSRD, corr. re Reports to President 1941-46 Box 2 "Science the Endless Frontier" Folder "General Committee #2." Letter J.E. Moore to Irwin Stewart.

67. NLMHMD Box nho Comments on S. 2721, Kilgore Bill to establish Off. Tech. Mobilization in letter from Surgeon General Parran to Asst. Genl. Counsel, FSA, December 14, 1942.

68. Archives of The National Academy of Sciences. Memorandum from the committee supporting the Bush report, 1945. Folder Executive Office for Emergency Management: OSRD 1944-45.

69. National Archives RG 227 OSRD, Office Chm NDRC and Dir. OSRD, corr. re Report to President 1941-1946; Box 1 "Science the Endless Frontier" Folder "Truman October 13, 45."

70. Archives of the National Academy of Sciences. Memorandum to signatories of letter to President Truman, December 1945. Folder Executive Office for Emergency Management: OSRD 1944-45.

71. S 1297 — Testimony of Dr. M. Demerec. Hearings on Science Legislation S 1297 and related bills, Parts 1-4, Oct 8 - Nov 2, 1945; Washington, DC.

72. Archives of The National Academy of Sciences. Memorandum from Homer Smith, undated. Folder: Executive Office for Emergency Management: OSRD, 1944-45.

73. Stewart I. p 320.

74. National Archives RG 227 OSRD Records of the CMR Box 32 General Records 1940-46. Folder "Dyer, R.E."

75. National Archives RG 227 OSRD Box 11 Minutes of the CMR, 1941-46. Folder: "September 6, 1945."

76. Hastings A.B. Personal communication.

77. National Archives NAHC Min .001. Minutes of joint NAHC/NACC meeting September 28, 1945.

78. Strickland. pp 21-50. Van Slyke, who was selected by Dyer to start the grants program, summarizes the start of the NIH Extramural Program.

79. Hearing Report Committee for Labor, FSA, and related independent offices appropriations, US House of Representatives; April 10, 1946; Washington, DC.

80. National Archives RG 443 Records of the National Institute of Health 1930-48. Res Grants. Box 1422. Folder "Research Grants Office."

81. Archives of The National Academy of Sciences. Annual Reports of the National Academy of Sciences, 1935 through 1948.
82. Data from Robert F. Moore, NIH DRG.
83. NIHCF file b&g 248. Memorandum from A.F. Siepert to the file, April 23, 1948. Meeting with FSA Program Planning Office.
84. Grob GN. The forging of mental health policy in America: World War II to New Frontier. *J Hist Med and Allied Studies*. 1987;42:6.
85. NLMHMD MS C 202 Box 22. Armstrong verification papers. Interview with Leonard Scheele by B.F. Armstrong.
86. Price DK. Endless Frontier or Bureaucratic Morass? *Daedalus*. 1978;107:75.
87. Kohler R.E. The Management of Science: The experience of Warren Weaver and the Rockefeller Foundation Program in Molecular Biology. *Minerva*. 1960;14:279-306.
88. Van Slyke CJ. New Horizons in Medical Research. *Science*. 1946;104:561.
89. NLMHMD MS C 203 George Rosen Collection of Oral History Transcripts. Interview with R.E. Dyer by Harlan Phillips. November 13, 1963.
90. Geiger RL. *To Advance Knowledge The Growth of American Research Universities 1900-1940*. New York, NY: Oxford University Press; 1986.
91. Executive Order 10521, signed by President Eisenhower on March 26, 1954; (CFR, Title 3 The President, 1954-1958 Compilation 183-185) empowered the NSF to review scientific programs of the federal government.
92. NLMHMD Records of the National Science Foundation's Special Committee on Medical Research, 1948-1975.
93. Kornberg A. *For the Love of Enzymes*. Boston, MA: Harvard University Press; 1989.
94. Corner GW. *A History of the Rockefeller Institute 1901-1950, Origins and Growth*. New York, NY: Rockefeller Institute Press; 1964.
95. In his book, *Ward 4*. Cambridge, MA: Harvard University Press; 1958, James Howard Means writes: "When research workers of the MGH visit Bethesda, Maryland and see the Clinical Center of the National Institutes of Health, they say 'Ah!, a 500-bed Ward 4.' "
96. In his cornerstone memoir (40), Thompson wrote: "I do not know of any other officer of my own times and I doubt if there will be many in the future to have the pleasure, excitement and good luck to be personally instrumental in the development of an institution such as the National Institutes of Health...."
97. Ralph C. Williams in his *The United States Public Health Service, 1788-1950*. Richmond, VA: Whittel & Shepperson; 1951), describes Thomas Parran's personal ranking of his considerable achievements. He gave the highest ranking to: first, the strengthening of the research programs of NIH and increasing extramural support of research; second, establishment of the NCI; and third, leadership of national venereal disease control. He was also a principal architect of the World Health Organization and responsible for the organization of the CDC.

CHAPTER II

Science, Technology, and Societal Goals

■ **Bondi H. Bridging the gulf.** *Technology in Society.* **1992;14:9-14.**

Reprinted with permission from Pergamon Press, Ltd.

Scientists and politicians have to work together in two different fields: (a) where a scientific input is required for sensible decision making by government ("science in policy"). (b) government support for science ("policy for science"). The very different background of scientists and of politicians makes cooperation difficult, particularly perhaps because of the very different time horizons of the two partners and the circumstance that, at least in academic life, scientists select their problems, whereas politicians inevitably have to deal with the problems that actually arise. To make the cooperation effective and fruitful, it is essential that the senior scientists involved should enjoy the confidence of the scientific community in general, should be able to convey the scientific knowledge, and especially the scientific uncertainties and doubts, with great lucidity to the politicians concerned, who although highly intelligent will only rarely have a scientific education, and that the scientific staff should be full members of the politician's team, conversant with what is politically feasible and what is not. As regards policy for science, it is important to be aware of the different reasons for public support of science: the cultural, the utilitarian and the educational.

. . . research is only considered successful and conveys fame on its author if it influences others, if it leads to further work. It is not important for the standing of the scientists that this further work should necessarily confirm all that has been said in the original paper. As long as it is stimulating, as long as a result of the discussion the [sic] knowledge and understanding increases and has been stimulated by the first work, then this deservedly has a high reputation. Generally in the performance of such research, time is not of the essence. As any researcher, but few other people know [sic], research is inevitably frustrating. One tries many different approaches before the problem shows the slightest signs of yielding, and very often the problem on which one actually makes one's contribution is somewhat different from the one on which one started.

Governing, the task of a politician, is quite different. The large majority of problems are not selected by the politician, they come upon the politician, and they may or may not be particularly amenable to intelligent analysis; but what is needed is an answer, a solution, and it is needed in a very limited time indeed.

The politician will be tied by colleagues, by party, by the overall policy of the government. What the politician hears in the discussion must be in a form that can be conveyed to and be impressed on colleagues. In 95% of cases scientists will be discussing an issue far beyond their own specialty in science.

We then come to a call for government to support science for a purpose. This may be military technology, it may be better materials for surfacing roads, it may be a better understanding of how pesticides work, or it may be a drug for diseases. In all these fields government should and ought to support science because it fits in with governmental purposes.

Lastly, there is the importance of science in education, in the education of people through doing science. Industry rightly looks to a large extent to government to supply the trained minds it needs to carry out its own purposes. An so in this field the purpose of government is not to create science, but to create *scientists*.

Science and government need each other. Their cooperation will be fruitful only if people with different backgrounds continuously work together in teams, jointly grappling with their common problems, each side bringing its own expertise to it, but fully sharing in the communal problem solving.

■ **Branscomb LM. Does America need a technology policy?** *Harvard Business Review.* **1992;70:24-28.**

From semiconductors to supercomputers, jumbo jets to HDTV, technology is probably the single most important factor driving the evolution of global competition. The accelerating pace of technological innovation is spawning new businesses, transforming old ones, and redefining the rules of competitive success.

Proponents of technology policy argue that a society's capacity for sustained technological innovation is crucial to its economic well-being. At a time when U.S. companies are steadily losing market share in strategic high-tech sectors, government support for R&D on "critical technologies" is absolutely essential.

Critics counter that however painful the loss of market share by U.S. companies might be, any governmental cure would be far worse than the disease.

The fact is, the issue isn't *whether* the United States should have a technology policy—it already does—but *what kind* of government policies and programs make sense in the new competitive environment.

For 40 years, an active federal government role in technology creation, diffusion, and adoption enjoyed a broad bipartisan consensus. This consensus engendered an implicit technology policy that decisively shaped patterns of technological innovation at U.S. companies.

This implicit technology policy consisted of two basic practices: generous government funding of basic research at universities and national laboratories and major investment by federal agencies in technology development directly related to their legally mandated missions. Policymakers assumed that government-funded science would benefit private industry by feeding a pipeline of innovation eventually leading to new technologies and whole new industries. And government-funded technology development, they reasoned, would spin off useful technology to the commercial sector.

This system worked reasonably well for more than 30 years.

What might a "capability enhancing" technology policy look like? Instead of focusing on picking winners, it would engage in activities that improve the overall innovative capacity of companies and the nation.

The closest the current debate comes to identifying such activities is in two other bits of policy jargon: "precompetitive" research on "generic" technologies.

As a guide to policy, this is unacceptably broad. But it does suggest one appropriate role for government: to support R&D that underpins a broad array of specific technology applications in many different industries, while stopping short of supporting proprietary technology that companies themselves should fund.

There are ways to encourage precompetitive R&D that do not involve spending public money. A big step would be to dismantle some of the many legal barriers blocking collaboration among companies and between companies, universities, and government labs.

■ **Carnegie Commission on Science, Technology, and Government.**
Enabling the Future: Linking Science and Technology to Societal
Goals. Washington, D.C.: Carnegie Commission on Science,
Technology, and Government, 1992.

In the next decade and those that follow, the United States will confront critical public policy issues that are intimately connected with advances in science and technology. Policy decision making will require the integration of numerous considerations, including accepted scientific knowledge, scientific uncertainty, and conflicting political, ethical, and economic values. Policy issues will not be resolved by citizens, scientists, business executives, or government officials working alone; addressing them effectively will require the concerted efforts of all sectors of society.

We believe that America faces a clear choice. For too long, our science and technology policies, apart from support of basic research, have emphasized short-term solutions while neglecting longer-term objectives. If this emphasis continues, the problems we have encountered in recent years, such as erosion of the nation's industrial competitiveness and the difficulties of meeting increasingly challenging standards of environmental quality, could overwhelm promising opportunities for progress. However, we believe there is an alternative. The United States could base its S&T policies more firmly on long-range considerations and link these policies to societal goals through more comprehensive assessment of opportunities, costs, and benefits.

Although this report touches on a number of goal-related themes, our recommendations focus on a few key issues: improving our national capacity to define and revise long-term S&T goals; linking S&T programs and goals more closely and clearly to broader societal goals; and building more effective linkages between governments (especially the federal government) and other sectors of society in debating, articulating, and pursuing these goals while assessing progress toward their achievement.

A nongovernmental National Forum on Science and Technology Goals should be established to facilitate the process of defining, debating, focusing, and articulating science and technology goals in the context of federal, national, and international goals, and to monitor the development and implementation of policies to achieve them.

Congress should devote more explicit attention to long-term S&T goals in its budget, authorization, appropriation, and oversight procedures.

In order to provide Congress with the information, analysis, and advice necessary to make policy decisions in this area, the Office of Technology Assessment and other congressional support agencies should evaluate national efforts to establish and achieve long-term science and technology goals in the context of societal goals.

The Office of Science and Technology Policy (OSTP) and the Office of Management and Budget (OMB) within the Executive Office of the President should actively contribute to the establishment of federal science and technology goals and should monitor the progress of departments and agencies in attaining these goals.

Federal departments and agencies should enhance their policy-making efforts, integrating considerations of long-term science and technology goals into annual budgeting and planning efforts.

■ **Cassman M. The evolution of a science advisory body in the federal government. *Perspectives in Biology and Medicine.* 1991;34:439-462.**

In 1940 the total federal expenditure for research and development was slightly less than $100 million. Most of these funds were for the conduct of science in government-owned installations, with the one significant exception being support of agriculture through the experimental stations. By 1948 federal support for R&D had reached $865 million, even after the termination of specific wartime programs such as the Manhattan Project. The time appeared uniquely suited to the achievement of a long-sought goal—the establishment of a centralized structure that would be responsible for all federally supported science, at least all basic research, and that could act as a central advisory body on science policy issues. The attempt to accomplish this failed, as had all previous attempts. The federal support of science remained as it had been from its earliest days—diffuse, diverse, and predominantly located in specific problem-oriented agencies.

Consequently, the problem of how to provide timely and readily accessible advice on issues related to science was, and still remains, of central importance, especially as it affects advice to the president.

For all of the nineteenth century and much of the early twentieth century, the major advisers to the government on science-related issues were the heads of agencies or bureaus. Not only did no one speak for all of science in the government, but the fragmentation of research within problem-oriented federal agencies, the antipathy to central functions as antidemocratic and elitist, and the absence of politically effective scientific organizations outside of government, all made the emergence of a broad advisory body highly unlikely.

It is clear that the need of the federal government for scientific advice beyond that available from the agencies emerged particularly during time of war, but the structures formed were often neglected after the emergency had passed.

It has frequently been noted that World War II transformed the relations of the scientific community and the federal government. It is equally remarkable that there was so little change in the institutional structures within which this transformation occurred.

Although the NSF [National Science Foundation] was empowered by statute to have a central coordinating and policy role in the federal science establishment, its comparatively minuscule budget reflected its real ability to execute these mandates. The advisory role was relegated to the individual agencies, according to their specific programmatic functions, and a multitude of other advisory committees were generated.

While this science advisory body was being established in the White House, congressional frustration was rising, as the members of Congress perceived that they were being shut out of an area of increasing importance, science policy. The NSF had not worked out as expected, becoming only another agency, somewhat weaker than most, rather than the center for all federal activities in R&D. Now a powerful new player had emerged: one sequestered in the White House, subject to executive privilege, and thus not responsive or accountable to Congress. But congressional needs remained unfulfilled, since perhaps the real urgency for such an agency was that it would generate a cabinet secretary who could appear before, and answer to, Congress.

In 1961, Jerome B. Wiesner, an MIT physicist, was named President Kennedy's science adviser. One of his first actions was to ask the PSAC [President's Science Advisory Committee] to examine the various proposals to strengthen the management and oversight of science in the federal government. The OST was established by executive order in 1962.

During Johnson's tenure, science was seen as just one more special-interest group, and Johnson saw the function of science in classic New Deal terms—as another mechanism to affect social politics. This view, together with accompanying populist attitudes, progressively alienated scientists and, with campus opposition to the Vietnam War, contributed to the decline of the adviser and PSAC, which reached its nadir during the Nixon era.

By now, however, the scientific community had a considerable emotional investment in the White House science office, along with a perhaps unjustified conviction that the office was a major factor in promoting their interests in Washington. Congress also was much distressed. As a result of these pressures and with the active encouragement of President Ford, a bill was passed in 1976 mandating an Office of Science and Technology Policy (OSTP) in the executive office of the president.

One of the peculiarities of OSTP over the years had been the limited involvement of the office with NIH and the life sciences generally.

Several reasons can be found for this phenomenon. First, NIH has always been seen as a creature of Congress. Successive administrations have struggled unsuccessfully to bring the NIH budget under the control of OMB and the White House.

This neglect of biomedical-related research and, by extension, of NIH, is changing radically with the emergence of the biotechnology industry, an industry that is a direct consequence of NIH investments in fundamental research in biology, chemistry, and even in some parts of physics.

In the absence of any such new jolt, it seems highly likely that a science advisory office to the President will remain what it is now, one of many federal entities that concern themselves with science. There are, in fact, those who feel that the current incarnation, the OSTP, is completely redundant, having neither the legislative authority to implement policy nor the intimate position in the White House to influence it. It is important, therefore, to consider again why such an office has ever been deemed necessary. Ultimately, it is to provide the President easy access to advice on issues of national importance in which science plays a role, independent of the institutional biases and conflicts that might color the contributions of the agencies.

Although the role of one among many is less grandiose than that of a science agency, it is more consistent with the pragmatic and decentralizing tendencies that have shaped the federal science establishment. The diversity of programs, agencies, and bureaus provides not one but many voices for science. It should be the primary goal of OSTP, or any presidential science advisory system, not to direct but to clarify and interpret this occasional cacophony, in aid of national policy.

■ **Curlin JW. Science and technology under constitutional separation of powers. *Technology in Society*. 1992;14:63-73.**

Reprinted with permission from Pergamon Press, Ltd.

Under the US Constitution, three bodies share equal authority for governance—the Executive, the Congress, and the Judiciary. Unlike parliamentary governments or authoritarian regimes, the President and the presidential advisors are but one element in the equation that determines U.S. policy. More often than not in the last 23 years, the President's party has been the minority party in Congress. Focussing attention solely on the Office of the President, as has been the tendency, ignores the reality that the Congress continues to be a major force for framing U.S. policy for science and technology. Congress has a workable analytical and advisory system for science and technology policy that meets its institutional needs. The executive branch, on the other hand, is still grappling with how factual, responsible, neutral analysis and advice can be effectively used in the politically charged atmosphere of the White House, where issues of science and technology often take a backseat to economic, political, and ideological considerations.

Experience in the United States suggests that a president who wants to get and use science advice will get and use science advice. The corollary is also true. The form and functions of the U.S. Government under the Constitution establish equals between President and Congress in the decision-making process; therefore we must have parallel science and technology advisory functions for the President and Congress. Under a parliamentary system, or where the legislature is weak relative to the power of the executive, a different science advisory apparatus might serve better.

Scientific and technical facts must be clearly separated from opinions and ideological bias. Neither can a science adviser be perceived as a protagonist of science for science's sake at the expense of balance and judgment. The best information is produced through competent neutrality by analysts who are intellectually equipped to assess the subject, while leaving the politics to others. This is not always easily achieved, particularly in the political atmosphere surrounding the President. It is more easily attained in a diversified, decentralized, bipartisan political environment like Congress.

No matter how large or competent the staff, valuable insights may be gained by involving the public in the analytical process. The pluralism of the U.S. culture ensures that there are many sides to issues of science and technology and many ways to view them.

Global environmental issues, transboundary telecommunications, transnational corporations, interlocked securities markets, and economic interdependency are current indicators of a world growing figuratively smaller and nations becoming more similar as a result of technology. The breadth of enquiry and analysis of science and technology issues must widen, as our national futures now depend as much on the actions of others as it does on our own determination.

■ **Newby H. One society, one Wissenschaft: a 21st century vision.** *Science and Public Policy.* **1992;19:7-14.**

Reprinted with permission of Beech Tree Publishing.

. . . the so-called "linear model" of how the natural sciences relate to social and economic progress. . . . begins with the view that scientific progress is itself exogenous to society. Basic science proceeds through a wholly innate process of scientific discovery. Such discoveries are then translated into various forms of technological change, and it is these changes in technology which provide the motor for social and economic progress.

But science alone does not change society: the history of the 20th century equally demonstrates that society can have a considerable impact on the nature of scientific activity.

. . . science has become much more like other institutions in modern society: in its organisational forms and work setting, in its moral standing and the norms held by its members, and in its affinity towards (some would say, corruption by) economic and political influence.

. . . the relationship between science, technology, and society is not uni-directional, as the linear model advocates, but is, in reality, interactive. Science changes society, but it is also socially constructed. Science enables technological development, but technological developments influence the course of science. Technology changes our everyday lives, but technology can only be developed where there is a market and where the products are socially acceptable or desirable.

. . . where science is closely linked to particular technological developments and to the design of public policy, it cannot be done credibly without a degree of co-operation from, and even collaboration with, representatives of the general public. At the very least, science must, to begin with, be transparent: that is, the uncertainties, assumptions and compromises underlying particular claims must be fully exposed to public scrutiny. This, of course, posits a new kind of relationship between science and the public.

The interactive model . . . . would place at centre stage the notion of innovation being driven by competition. Such competitive innovation is in turn continually evaluated by the prevailing market environment, which appears as an active and variable element, both shaping and being shaped by technological change.

. . . social science is an integral, and not merely a marginal, activity in understanding the process whereby scientific excellence and technological inno-vation may lead to economic and social well-being. For this to be effective, social science investigation should not be restricted to the down-stream study of impacts and diffusion, but should be integrated into the study of the very processes themselves. Social and natural scientists have complementary skills, and mutual interests, in together improving the processes of technological innovation. This will involve a degree of multi-disciplinarity, if not inter-disciplinarity, which spans not only the social sciences but transcends the two cultures.

■ Owen D. **Improving the input of scientific advice into political decision making.** *Technology in Society.* **1992;14:37-47.**

Reprinted with permission from Pergamon Press, Ltd.

The scientist can be an uneasy, but very useful adviser to the politician. Yet if science is to guide government more effectively a quantum leap in openness is needed. Scientists, like anyone else, have views, interests, and prejudices that affect their work and advice. One example is that negotiations towards a Comprehensive Nuclear Test Ban Treaty have been effectively frustrated by scientists since 1977. Scientific advances can, even in normal circumstances, take a decade to enter public policy. Another example quoted is the AIDS pandemic which has met prejudice sufficient to overthrow good public health practice. The rejection of routine blood testing, despite its proven success in dealing with syphilis a century earlier, will be looked back upon as a monumental error of judgment. Flexible realistic mechanisms are put forward for improving the input of scientific advice into political decision making.

All heads of government should personally appoint the chair of a Scientific Advisory Council. The Council should be formed from eminent scientists from the varied scientific disciplines. The chair should not become a full-time government employee, but preferably be seconded from their [sic] place of employment for a specified period and have, if they wish, time to continue on a part-time basis with that employment. This will ensure their independence.

The Council should be multi-disciplinary, drawn from scientists within and outside government.

The Council should aim to encourage scientific debate in areas related to government decision making. It would cover all aspects of policy, and defence would not be excluded. In most cases the Council's deliberations could be made public.

The Scientific Advisory Council should, as well as looking forward, also look back. There are great potential benefits from the medical practice of conducting postmortems to discover what went wrong and what went right.

International meetings of the heads of each country's scientific advisory Council should be encouraged, and there would be value in exchanging documentation between councils.

■ **Task Force on the Health of Research.** *Chairman's Report to the Committee on Science, Space, and Technology, U.S. House of Representatives, One Hundred Second Congress.* **Washington, D.C.: U.S. Government Printing Office, 1992.**

This report outlines broad strategies by which the Committee on Science, Space, and Technology (SST) can strengthen its oversight of the federally funded research portfolio, while crafting policy to improve the linkages between federally funded research programs and national goals such as energy security, environmental protection, innovation in high technology manufacturing, expanding the knowledge base, and educating future scientists and engineers. The report is not intended to be comprehensive; rather, it seeks to expand the current science policy dialogue, which has been too narrowly focused on funding levels, and not sufficiently concerned with the structure of the research system.

The Task Force on the Health of Research views national goals as the motivating force behind federal support for research. This perspective suggests two lines of analysis that must underlie federal research policy:

(1) For a given national goal, what research is most necessary?

(2) How can we best conduct such research? That is, what mechanisms for administering, performing, and evaluating research create the optimal pathways from research to goal attainment?

To answer these questions, the Committee will need to examine and evaluate traditional science policy assumptions and recommend new approaches; expand the range of experts upon whom it calls for advice to include the users of research, rather than just the performers; and establish programs that compare and assess alternative methods of research administration and performance. In this context, the Task Force recommends two nested lines of actions aimed at creating more explicit linkages between national goals and federally supported research programs:

(1) Strengthen mechanisms for setting government-wide research-policy goals, and for oversight of the federal research portfolio, by exploiting Committee jurisdiction over the Office of Science and Technology Policy;

(2) Integrate performance assessment mechanisms into the research process using legislative mandates and other measures, to help measure the effectiveness of federally funded research programs.

Implementating the recommendations of this report will require a long term, strategic approach by the Committee that will probably include hearings, pilot projects, and legislative initiatives embracing the jurisdictions of most or all of the SST subcommittees. The report itself is not a detailed recipe; rather, it is designed to serve as the starting point of a constructive dialogue and evolutionary process that can strengthen the Committee's ability to forge science policy for the national good.

David R. Challoner

T hat din you hear outside of your window does indeed indicate a jam on the traffic circle of science policy. It has been caused by the coming together in the same intersection at this moment in time of a variety of historic political changes in society and evolutionary or developmental events in science. Among these changes are the end of the Cold War as a logic for significant societal investment in defense-related research, a disquiet in the science community created by an increasing discrepancy between the number of scientists and the resources needed to support their inquiries, and a society which has lost faith in science as a controlling factor in the resolution of our problems with the environment, AIDS, and economic competitiveness.

Western societies, through their governments, are looking for answers to these problems and are increasingly questioning the linear theory which has predominated in explaining the benefits of basic research to society since World War II—that is, the societal technological applications flow naturally and unidirectionally from a heavy investment in fundamental research. Rather, some research and policy analysts such as Howard Newby are studying the multiple feedback loops on the pathway from insight to output and seeking to control the traffic in ways other than simply putting greater or lesser resources into basic research.

Thus, we are poised for a major rethinking of the relationship of fundamental research to societal well-being and the subsequent development of government policies to facilitate this process. Over the next decade, this will affect all of us. Scientists and the institutions in which they work will be affected, and the relationship with government sponsors may change in dramatic ways similar to the setting of the paradigm that followed World War II and lasted half a century. Biomedicine, the life sciences, and our institutions, must be prepared for some discomfort in these changes.

The articles selected for this chapter of the third health policy annual, *Science, Technology, and Societal Goals*, provide an excellent "primer" on these issues by important participants in the debate. The issues raised are necessary to understanding the debate. I recommend them to you. All of the relevant institutional players in the research game are currently and actively involved in describing their part of the elephant, to wit:

- The Executive Branch, through the President's Council of Advisors on Science and Technology and the Office of Science and Technology Policy, under the guidance of the White House Science Advisor, has just released reports on the research universities and technology transfer.
- The Legislative Branch, through Congressman Brown's Committee on Science, Space and Technology, has just released a report of the Task Force on the Health of Research.
- The federal science agencies are carrying out their own analyses, including the National Science Foundation's (NSF) recent report on the future of the NSF and the National Institutes of Health's (NIH) strategic plan.
- The scientific community is gearing up for reports from the American Association for Advancement of Science and from specialty areas such as astrophysics, where true priority setting was attempted.
- The universities, through the Association of American Universities, have studied a variety of these issues, including indirect costs.
- Industry has pursued an understanding of the process through the Government Industry University Round Table and other such activities.
- The public interest has been pursued by foundations such as Carnegie as represented by its Commission Report.
- The academy complex (National Academy of Science, National Academy of Engineering, Institute of Medicine, and National Research Council) is currently striving to understand the changing paradigm through its horizon-scanning Committee on Science,

Engineering and Public Policy and to set a course for the next several decades as the Vannevar Bush Report did for the latter half of the 20th century.

Thus, this is not a passing phase in science policy to be disregarded by those of us concerned with the life sciences and their application, but rather it is a debate in which we must be informed participants.

It is interesting that the life sciences have been relatively isolated from this sort of policy oversight and from related decision-making and advisory structures, in particular in the executive branch, which have monitored other fields of science. As pointed out by Marvin Cassman, the life sciences' primary government patron has been the National Institutes of Health. The NIH is more a creature of Congress than the Executive Branch agencies, such as the Department of Defense, which oversee the rest of science. As a result, the life sciences have developed without the same sponsor-driven policy oversight other than a conviction in the Congress that they must be good for the health of the public. The bioscience community was able to maintain support for an investigator-initiated basic science paradigm as nearly the *sole* device to get there. Congress was not in a position to question their bioscience offspring until now.

A second outcome of this unique history is that the various umbrella policy-making bodies and advisory groups in the Executive Branch, such as the President's Council of Advisors on Science and Technology, the National Science Board in the NSF, and even some of the policy committees in the National Academy of Sciences, find the life sciences significantly under-represented in relation to the proportion of the federal research effort now devoted to the life sciences. This policy weakness in the biosciences has become increasingly apparent as items such as the importance of biotechnology to industrial competitiveness and the technology-driven problem of health care costs have risen to public attention, not even considering all the other matters of societal concern outlined in the introduction to this commentary. It is imperative that representatives of the life sciences and the academic health centers in which they are housed be involved in these discussions relative to their participation in the overall scientific enterprise. In this instance, we cannot depend on the NIH or our congressional sponsors to carry the water.

Our nation's academic health centers and their parent universities have a significant stake in this fascinating, outcome-oriented policy discussion. These institutions are the sites that produce most of our life science research, a modicum of development to socially useful products, and educate almost all of the scientific manpower to carry on the entire process.

The articles in this chapter are recommended to the reader because they give a broad view across the entire spectrum of science and its relation to the society which supports it. We cannot afford to take the narrow view, or we will not be credible players. This narrow view has been exposed by the heated defense of the investigator-initiated grant numbers in the political process and in the negative reaction of many of the life science societies to the Institute of Medicine's report on the importance of including human and fixed capital infrastructure in the funding policies for biomedical research. It is hoped that this volume will create some understanding of the expanded scope of the discussion that is upon us. I recommend it to you.

COMMENTARY

Ralph Snyderman

The benefits of science and technology have the potential to alleviate many societal problems in the areas of health care, environmental protection, energy security, and national economic competitiveness. Given the magnitude of and heightened awareness about these issues, an imperative is developing to create an overall strategy regarding federal funding for science and technology. Of the government's $75 billion investment in science and technology in FY '93, about $15 billion are allocated for biomedically related research. Substantial financial support for science and technology began in earnest during World War II in response to national defense needs for military purposes and health protection. Funding for biomedical research associated with an invigorated and expanding National Institutes of Health grew rapidly in the 1960s and was followed by moderate real growth. However, funding levels did not grow in real terms for the first time this past year. While federal funding of science and technology has been a subject of ongoing debate for decades, this topic has become the subject of heightened discussion during the past two years. A basic question being asked is whether federal expenditures for science and technology could be more wisely invested. It is likely that changes in policy will occur, but the nature and timing of the changes are uncertain.

Federal funding for biomedical research was based on the assumption that the investment would result in broad societal good. The policies that governed such funding were not strategically formed and apparently based on the concept that basic biomedical research, as a source of freely available knowledge, would eventually lead to useful applications. Furthermore, it has been assumed that investigator-initiated research was likely to be the most creative type of research, that peer review enhanced the value of the investment, and that most research would occur in academic or federal research institutions. Historically, commercialization of basic research discoveries in academia was driven by industrial surveillance of such research. More recently, academicians, academic institutions, and governmental research entities have been encouraging and facilitating technology transfer. This is not to say that there has not been overall direction of biomedical research towards practical application. For example, each of the National Institutes of Health is disease-oriented, and research within the intramural and extramural programs of the National Institutes of Health is more or less balanced in its application to problems raised by prevalent diseases. Nonetheless, there has been heightened concern recently that the generally "bottoms-up" strategy of federally funded, basic biomedical research (i.e., investigator initiated) is not sufficiently meeting national health or economic needs.

No coherent national policy for science and technology, in general, and for biomedical research, in particular, appears to exist. Focusing on the latter, oversight occurs within numerous federal agencies, including the Office of Science and Technology Policy (OSTP), the Federal Coordinating Council on Science Engineering and Technology (FCCSET), the Office of Management and Budget (OMB), several congressional committees, including the House Committee on Science, Space, and Technology, and within such departments as Health and Human Services, Defense, and Agriculture. Many arguments can be made that the federal investment in science and technology has paid untold dividends, with much more ready to unfold, and that changes to the system could do more harm than good. Even so, debates in this area are inevitable and could well lead to more stable funding for basic research and better mechanisms for efficient translation of research discoveries into practical applications.

Responding to the imperatives for strategic planning, several initiatives have begun. Under the leadership of Bernadine Healy, M.D., director of the National Institutes of Health, a long-range strategic plan was developed for biomedical research. The Committee on Science Based Technology of the U.S. House of Representatives has developed a report of the Task Force on the Health of Research (Chairman's Report to the Committee on Science, Space, and Technology), which clearly identifies a need for a national policy. The purpose of such a policy would be "to improve the linkages between federally funded research programs and national goals such as energy security, environmental protection, innovation in high technology manufacturing, expanding the knowledge base, and educating future scientists and engineers." The thoughtful report of this committee suggests two lines of analysis to underlie federal research policy. "One, for a given national goal, what research is most necessary? Two, how can we best conduct such research? That is, what mechanisms for administering, performing, and evaluating research create the optimal pathways from research to goal attainment?" This committee is suggesting that rather than relying on the assumption that funding outstanding research will ultimately benefit the nation, one needs a strategic plan that starts with national objectives and works back towards the mechanisms by which to achieve them. Given the fact that federal funding of research must be expected to be worthwhile and cost effective, it is only reasonable that the federal government should play a role in determining whether it is getting full value for its investment. What must be determined is whether a new or different policy would more efficiently translate federal biomedical research expenditures into benefits for society.

Change from the current model to a more highly planned national model is not a trivial issue since the present system, with all its faults and inefficiencies, has led to explosive advances in our understanding of biology, the effective treatment and prevention of many diseases, and the emerging biotechnology revolution. The current system has placed us on the threshold of previously unimagined opportunities for improving human health. While the development of new policy appears to be inevitable, changes should be made cautiously lest they upset the fragile structures of basic science that underpin our nation's (and indeed the world's) magnificent biomedical research enterprise.

To develop a national plan for biomedical research and the applications to societal good, one must define the objectives to be achieved. General goals have been identified by the Report of the Task Force on the Health of Research. They are a useful starting point. These goals are "achieving national energy security, enhancing environmental protection, improving health, increasing the productivity and profitability of high technology industries, maintaining a healthy research infrastructure, expanding a knowledge base, educating future scientists, and creating a scientifically and technologically literate work force."

How then do we fashion a national policy to meet these goals? In my view the establishment of more specific national goals, objectives, and priorities, and the creation of a rational governing structure for oversight, development, and implementation of a plan are needed as well as a mechanism for appropriate funding and monitoring of progress and outcome. To accomplish these ends, we must first understand more fully how the current system permits basic research discoveries to produce practical applications. We must identify and understand what functions well and what barriers limit the current system. We must understand the degree to which non-directed, basic, unfocused research underpins any successful applications model. This is a formidable task and is, in my opinion, among the most important initial requirements for the development of a national science and technology policy.

A suggested means for defining and understanding the current system would be to identify a number of important advances in clinical care and to determine the pathways by which they developed from the initial ideas and research discoveries to successful application. A model for this type of analysis was provided by Comroe and Dripps in their study of successful applications in the areas of pulmonary and cardiovascular medicine.[1] I would propose broadening this type of study to include classical pharmaceutical agents, vaccines, biotechnology products, devices, and instruments. It is important to determine as specifically as possible how fundamental, curiosity-driven research fosters basic, biologically related research. This research then advances disease-related research and enhances research with clinical application which finally results in the development of clinical applications.

It is not likely that the model for development of useful pharmaceutics or vaccines is the same as the development of useful biotechnology products or complex diagnostic or therapeutic instruments. It is also important to determine how the increasing pace and effectiveness of biotechnology as well as the heightened understanding of biological processes are changing the way "unfocused" research can be translated to practical use.

A large pool of unstructured, unfocused, investigator-initiated, basic research will undoubtedly underlie any subsequent commercial application. Policymakers should understand, and incorporate this idea in any strategic biomedical science and technology plan. There is less agreement about the amount and types of unstructured basic research which are necessary to ensure continued development of successful application. What remains to be determined is the amount of federal support that should go into such research versus other areas of research and development and the degree to which the government should participate in the financial rewards from successful applications.

Given the nation's $900 billion of investment, it is not unreasonable to spend at least $15 billion (1.7 percent) for the direct and indirect costs of biomedical research and the development and training of future scientists. Indeed, a substantialy larger, more strategic investment could well be justified since industry generally spends more than 10 percent of its expenses on Research & Development. In any case, a substantial pool of research that is not related to disease will be necessary to sustain the advancement of medical progress. It is very likely that the federal government will be the only stable provider of sufficient funds for such research and its infrastructure.

In the construction of any plan to change the current system, a number of tensions will need to be specifically assessed. These will include the role of federal funding for a variety of research categories, including unfocused, curiosity-driven research, biological process or disease-related research, and disease-modifying research. Additional questions concerning research funding include: (1) the value of classical reductionist approaches to problem solving versus holistic approaches. There appears to be mounting political pressure for the latter although the former has a proven track record of success.; (2) the benefit of peer review for research quality versus review for societal impact and review for political purposes; (3) the value of investigator-initiated versus government-initiated research; (4) the amount of funding needed for research infrastructure and the training of future scientists of various types; (5) the impact of encouraging focused research on the quality of fundamental research discoveries; and (6) the effect of commercialization on the academic nature of universities and non-commercial research institutes.

Where do we go from here? Sir Francis Bacon states, "Truth

springs more quickly from error than from confusion." We would be best served by having some appropriate group develop descriptive models of how the current research system works (with all its strengths and flaws) and specific proposals for improved models for the translation of fundamental research to practical application that would include the role of federal funding. I would charge this group with addressing, as specifically as possible, the nature of how the "hand-offs" in this current system occur and how this process might be improved. This group in conjunction with perhaps another more politically oriented body could overlay the model with suggested national priorities, governance mechanisms, and funding strategies. For the first part, I would suggest that the Congress charge the Institute of Medicine to conduct a comprehensive study to define the real value of basic research in terms of societal benefit and to develop concrete models useful to more rational strategic planning.

Some strategic questions to be addressed include the following:

(1) What are the goals, objectives, and priorities for federally funded research? (2) How does the government maximize the effectiveness of this funding (i.e. its return on investment)? (3) What is appropriate level of funding for research and development and their infrastructure? (4) How should funding be distributed among areas of research and development from unfocused-discovery research through applied development research? (5) How does government determine value of this investment over time?

This report could be reviewed by the OSTP or a committee assembled by this office to deal with the development of a preliminary National Science and Technology Research Policy. This proposal would be subject to broad review by the appropriate constituencies and ultimately refined into legislation by Congress through its appropriate subcommittees.

With all its flaws, the current system has achieved magnificent advances in science and technology and has allowed the United States to lead the world in this area. Indeed, the entire world is dependent upon this nation's scientific research enterprise. Policymakers must understand how any new policy could disrupt this successful yet fragile system and the potential risks for significantly harming the current system. With these cautions in mind, the development of a rational national strategic plan could be a great aid in enhancing the efficiency and cost effectiveness of federal funding of science and technology.

Summary. The development of a more focused national policy for science and technology funding is needed and will likely occur. Under the current system, the federal government now invests about $15 billion per year in biomedical research. It is an investment that has enabled tremendous advances in our understanding of biology and disease as well as in medical therapeutics. Nonetheless, there is no coherent strategic policy, and for planning purposes a better understanding of what works and what does not work in the current system is needed.

There is a growing debate to suggest that federally funded research should be more closely linked to fulfilling national health and economic needs. Many scientists are concerned that such discussions could lead to a diminution of support for fundamental, investigator-initiated biomedical research as a consequence of funding politically appealing, short-sighted goals. What is not well understood is how much non-applied, discovery research funding is needed to sustain a continued flow of application research and development. The establishment of a strategic plan, including more specific national goals and objectives for federally funded biomedical research could enhance the public support of research funding. In addition, the effectiveness of the research enterprise in translating its discoveries into cost-effective health care and national economic viability would also be enhanced. However, it must be understood that in any plan, a strong foundation of basic "non-directed" research will be required for all that follows. It would be useful for a group such as the Institute of Medicine or some other prestigious organization to be charged with the development of a preliminary strategic plan.

Reference

1. Comroe JH Jr, Dripps RD. Scientific basis for the support of biomedical science. *Science.* 1976;192:105-111.

Setting Priorities and Allocating Funds for Biomedical Research

---

ABSTRACTS AND EXCERPTS

■ **Brennan TA. Government and science: stimulation or inhibition. *Bull NY Acad Med*. 1992;68:151-161.**

Reprinted with permission, courtesy of the New York Academy of Medicine.

. . . it is often overlooked that the conduct of molecular biology research raises a series of questions about science policy and the funding of investigations. Scientific research can be underwritten by multiple sources, each generating different goals and expectations. As a result, investigators can face a series of conflicts of interest, and policy makers must make choices about appropriate funding mechanisms. Moral and political considerations raised by the financing of research are no less real than the more frequently discussed dilemmas arising out of care for individual patients.

The Human Genome Project is in many ways a new method for funding biological research, and it is controversial. The perception of many is that the Human Genome Project will provide block grants for particular groups of researchers, creating largesse among favored investigators; meanwhile most other laboratories can expect diminished levels of funding.

From a science policy viewpoint, the important question about the Project remains: will it provide the most expedient path to greatest knowledge at least cost? Answering this question requires an institutional analysis, taking into account relationships between the various loci for medical research, especially academic institutions and pharmaceutical firms. In particular, we want to know whether the focussed approach of the Human Genome Project, the designation of funds for a specific project to well-defined centers, identifies and ameliorates the conflicts of interest that can arise in the pursuit of research better than does the decentralized funding strategy of the traditional RO1 grants.

The Genome Project would appear to contribute to useful consideration of university-pharmaceutical conflicts in two ways. First, the Human Genome Project itself provides large grants to specific laboratories, presumably making them somewhat independent of the need for "for-profit" funding. These laboratories can pursue their projects with some freedom; they need not find successful market-place applications of discoveries. Second, Project results will be available to all members of the public, including industry. This will dampen the concerns of those fearful that the independence of academic researchers and the public availability of the information they produce will be hampered by the influence of for-profit concerns in medical research.

Potential conflict between physician researchers and patients for whom they care could be an even greater source of ethical problems than conflicts between academic and for-profit values.

The relative interests of patients whose body parts might give rise to biotechnology products and of researchers who may seek profit from such products must be weighed carefully by courts. . . . the Project will want to set an example of informed consent and commitment to research subject welfare in the projects it funds.

. . . the Project's policy of free access to technology it develops should co-exist happily with a policy of allowing patents for biotechnology companies.

The Project's leadership should address concerns of science funding and the conflicts of interest generated by for-profit enterprise. The end result should be policy development that is rational and provides the best possible path to the potentially revolutionary results of genetic research.

■ Friedman H. Big science vs. little science: the controversy mounts. *Cosmos.* 1991;1:8-14.

In the current turmoil over the federal budget there are ominous portents for the scientific endeavor. Many research activities may be forced to shrink and an emotional debate is already underway about how the squeeze should be applied across the spectrum of small and big science. In every field, sponsors are emphasizing *directed* research that can make early contributions to economic productivity, human benefits and the solution of environmental problems.

From its head start in the war years, big science has dominated the scientific enterprise with an ever-escalating growth. But there are many scientists who still view small, undirected science, motivated purely by the researcher's curiosity to unlock the secrets of nature, as the wellspring from which technological revolutions grow.

Big science is here to stay. For the most part, the science is well conceived if not always ideally executed. We need to seek improvement, not attrition, and big-science management must be challenged not to repeat the tragic mistakes of the Hubble telescope.

What is worrisome now is that a substantial growth in recent years of the number of scientists working on small science is not being matched by increasing grant support from the scientific agencies. Unless the trend toward severe austerity is corrected, many promising young scientists will be forced to seek their livelihoods in other professions—and American sciences will suffer.

■ Institute of Medicine. *Research and Service Programs in the PHS: Challenges in Organization.* Washington, D.C.: National Academy Press, 1991.

Over the past 25 years, a number of attempts have been made to reform the organizational structure of the Public Health Service (PHS). The expressed goals of reorganizations include increasing efficiency and economy, promoting more effective planning and coordination, and reducing fragmentation or overlap. The reorganizations have also had political goals.

This study responds to a congressional requirement in the Anti-Drug Abuse Act of 1988 (P.L. 100-690) that the Secretary of Health and Human Services request the National Academy of Sciences to conduct a review of the research activities of NIH, ADAMHA, and related agencies. Specifically, the committee was asked for:

- an evaluation of the appropriateness of administering health service programs in conjunction with the administration of biomedical and behavioral research; and
- a determination of the extent of duplication among selected research programs of NIH and ADAMHA.

Lack of clarity about the services mission of the PHS seems to be a more important factor than organizational structure in problems relating to the administration of services development and demonstration (treatment or prevention) programs. . . . the committee recommends that the Secretary further clarify the services mission of the PHS and of the agencies that administer programs related to development of the structure and delivery of services. Services programs should be given stability, including stability of organizational location, financing, personnel, and other resources. The committee recommends that the Assistant Secretary for Health take responsibility for assessing and enhancing the integration of program objectives related to the services mission across agencies in the PHS.

The committee recommends that below the agency level, research and services programs be administered and conducted by separate institutes or offices that have substantial expertise in the specific substantive and functional area.

The committee encountered no persuasive evidence that overwhelmingly supports any specific agency structure, and it therefore recommends that agency-level organization not be used as the basis for deterring or encouraging reorganization. If reorganization of current agency structure is considered, it should be justified purely on policy grounds.

The committee recommends that replication, which is vital to basic and clinical research but which has not been considered a central element of demonstrations, be ensured in new and ongoing research demonstrations following single-site experiments and prior to implementation and national dissemination.

. . . the committee recommends that a research program be initiated within the PHS to determine effective dissemination mechanisms for demonstrations and the results of health services research.

The committee recommends that a plan for incentives for translation of successful demonstration findings into the structure and delivery of services be accompanied by opportunities for state review and comment on all types of federal demonstration applications.

The committee recommends that the responsibility for technical assistance and clinical training programs for professionals and nonprofessionals, and the resources to carry them out, be part of the explicit mission of agencies that fund and administer operating programs (e.g., HRSA, the Indian Health Service, and ADAMHA).

■ Kirschner M. The need for unity in the biomedical research community. *Academic Medicine*. 1991;66:577-582.

Reprinted with permission of *Academic Medicine* (formerly the *Journal of Medical Education*).

The author provides a perspective on how basic scientists view contemporary issues of biomedical research funding by discussing five topics of concern to the biomedical research community and the need for that community to form a new consensus as the basis for new approaches to legislative efforts in Congress and communication with the public. The topics are (1) the reasons scientific societies became active in legislative efforts in Congress, (2) the reasons there was initial friction between these societies and other institutions in the biomedical research community, (3) the history of the founding of a biomedical research caucus in the House of Representatives, (4) the effects of the Institute of Medicine's recent report on funding health sciences research, and (5) the weakness of the present institutional coalition. The author proposes specific steps to develop a more unified approach to achieve a common biomedical research agenda.

What is needed is a new means of bringing scientists and administrators, along with representatives from voluntary health organizations, together to plan both the long-term strategy and the short-term tactics.

How do we assemble a consensus and how do we put our aims into effect? For long-term planning we must assemble leaders of science and institutions into several small groups to deal with issues such as management of the NIH, legislative agendas, indirect costs, training plans, conflict of interest, and ethics in science.

For short-term tactical policy on legislation, we need a standing committee of selected scientists, administrators, and voluntary health workers. . . . [to] forge a common approach across the entire biomedical community.

On the most immediate level, scientific societies and institutional groups must work together in our approach to congressional committees.

■ National Institutes of Health. The "Strategic Plan": mixing salesmanship and science. *The Journal of NIH Research*. 1992;4:33-40.

Reprinted with permission from *The Journal of NIH Research*.

NIH Director Bernadine Healy is on a mission. It is to lay out a "strategic plan" for U.S. biomedical science and NIH unlike anything before it.

Healy unveiled the much-heralded strategic plan—recast from the original 1991 draft as a "framework for discussion of strategies for the NIH"—at a large gathering of federal and extramural scientists in San Antonio at the beginning of February [1992].

By the third meeting in Atlanta, however, most researchers attending the meeting appeared convinced that a strategic plan is a political necessity. Their abiding skepticism centered on worries that the plan would be implemented top-down and, most especially, that any research not linked somehow to a designated critical technology, public health need, or a return on investment would be unlikely to get federal funding.

Only two things about the strategic plan are certain, Healy and other NIH officers told the scientists. First, there will be a strategic plan, and second, NIH will begin to package funding requests to Congress differently—in terms of scientific programs and opportunities rather than numbers of grants.

Assurances from NIH institute directors notwithstanding, many feared that R01s might be an endangered species.

As a political marketing tool, the strategic plan that emerges from all this will have to be concise, easy to understand, and persuasive. If it is to reflect the needs and priorities of the scientific community, it will have to be flexible.

If researchers were determined that basic research should not bow to commercial or public health exigencies, they were no less concerned about seeing to it that basic research is translated into clinical medicine. The link, many said, is the physician-scientist, who—though not yet a missing link—is surely a rare find in today's economy.

Just as the M.D.-Ph.D. can straddle two realms, so too can the general clinical research centers serve as the natural meeting ground for basic and clinical research—but not if they remain so underfunded that they are equipped for little more than urinalysis, . . .

Researchers who attended the meetings expressed feelings ranging from distaste to outright alarm at the intrusion of "economic competitiveness" into deliberations on the merits of scientific research.

The first of the proposed NIH goals in the framework document—"to foster innovative research strategies"—garnered the heartiest endorsements. It also provoked the loudest cries that much of the proposed strategic plan in fact thwarted that goal with "micromanagement" and prescriptive research-priority lists.

Most of all, most extramural scientists said they want a strategic plan that is flexible, that reflects their collective judgments, and that doesn't damn valuable research by faint or no praise.

■ **National Institutes of Health.** *The Status of Biomedical Research Facilities: 1990.* **Washington, D.C.: U.S. DHHS, 1991.**

The size, condition, and adequacy of research facilities affect the nation's ability to conduct research. To obtain systematic and reliable data on the status of research facilities, Congress directed the National Science Foundation (NSF), in the Authorization Act (P.L. 99-159, section 108):

. . . to design, establish, and maintain a data collection and analysis capability . . . for the purpose of identifying and assessing the research facilities needs of universities and colleges . . . The Foundation, in conjunction with other appropriate Federal agencies, shall conduct the necessary surveys every 2 years and report the results to the Congress.

This report is based upon NSF's 1990 Survey of Scientific and Engineering Research Facilities at Universities and Colleges. This survey was the second full-scale study involving research space by science/engineering field and type of institution.

This report, reflecting the co-sponsorship of the survey by the National Institutes of Health, focuses specifically on biomedical research facilities, and includes nonprofit research organizations and independent hospitals as well as the academic institutions covered in the earlier report.

Of a total 186 million net assignable square feet of space assigned to biomedical disciplines in 1990, 55 million square feet (30 percent) was devoted to organized research. This was an increase from 52 million NASF in 1988. The space was primarily located at medical schools (42 percent) and colleges and universities (41 percent); . . .

Biomedical research space increased by 13 percent at public colleges and universities, but decreased by 13 percent at private colleges and universities. At medical schools, biomedical research space increased by 7 percent in both public and private institutions.

. . . a sizable minority (41 percent) reported *inadequate* research space.

Space was most often judged *inadequate* at medical schools (57 percent) and colleges and universities (44 percent), . . .

Little change occurred overall in perceptions of adequacy between 1988 and 1990, but some changes occurred in specific disciplines or institutional settings.

The rising construction expenditures from 1986-87 to 1988-89 were due entirely to a growth in the amount of space under construction, since unit costs remained stable at $258 per square foot for new construction.

Despite the stability in total expenditures for repair/renovation, the unit costs increased with each successive time period, and the amount of space being renovated decreased.

The increase in needed but deferred repair/renovation was due both to a decrease in the amount of space planned for repair/renovation in 1990-91 and to a projected increase in unit costs.

The primary sources of funds for new construction of biomedical research facilities were state/local governments, private donations, institutional funds, and debt financing.

Public and private institutions were substantially different in their sources of new construction funding. Public colleges and universities received more than half of their funding from state and local governments, and public medical schools received one-third of their funding from these sources. In comparison, private institutions received 1 percent or less from state and local governments, instead receiving funds primarily from private donations and debt financing.

Institutional funds were the primary source for funding repair/renovation projects, especially for private institutions.

■ **National Institutes of Health.** *Framework for Discussion of Strategies for NIH.* **Washington, D.C.: U.S. Department of Health and Human Services, 1992.**

The biomedical and behavioral sciences have entered an era of unprecedented opportunity, a new age of discovery and application. Much of this progress is attributable to NIH's sustained support for fundamental biology and clinical research. To ensure that this momentum will go forward and that the past Federal investment in biomedical research will continue to be capitalized, NIH has been engaged in a synergistic process involving all its organizational components, as well as ADAMHA and its research institutes, to develop a framework for discussion of strategies to guide the NIH as it advances into the 21st century. This "framework" identifies and advances activities that we view to be of strategic importance to the success of the enterprise as it impacts on the public's health and the nation's economy into the 21st century. It has a scope that transcends immediate interests and is responsive to changing public and national health needs. Importantly, it builds on past accomplishments, organizational strengths, and mechanisms and approaches of proven value. Finally, it creates a framework for focussing NIH's corporate thinking and charts an initial course for our efforts.

As part of this "framework for discussion" we have developed a mission statement, goals, and underlying principles for the agency. . . . This unifying corporate philosophy articulates a shared vision of how the biomedical research enterprise and the science it supports will advance.

Anchoring this framework are broad trans-NIH objectives which relate to specific operational components. . . . While the objectives are interrelated, and therefore cannot be placed in rank order, they represent the context within which the entire framework for discussion should be considered.

OBJECTIVE 1 — CRITICAL TECHNOLOGIES

Assure that critical technologies in basic biology impacting on human health and the national economy are advanced as priorities across the NIH.

OBJECTIVE 2 — RESEARCH CAPACITY

Strengthen the capacity of the national biomedical and behavioral research enterprise to respond to current and emerging public health needs.

OBJECTIVE 3 — INTELLECTUAL CAPITAL

Provide for the renewal and growth of the intellectual capital base essential to the biomedical research enterprise. Ensuring fairness and equality of opportunity at NIH is central to efforts to enhance the human resource base of biomedical research.

OBJECTIVE 4 — STEWARDSHIP OF PUBLIC RESOURCES

Secure the maximal return on the public investment in the enterprise.

OBJECTIVE 5 — PUBLIC TRUST

Continually earn the public's respect, trust, and confidence as we carry out our mission.

The strategic planning process charts a course for those efforts that are critical to the success of the entire enterprise.

A strategic plan is not a static document or an event, but rather a dynamic process that will evolve over time and use.

The implementation phase of a strategic plan will be guided by the following principles:

1. *The Institutes, Centers and Divisions (ICDs) are the Agents for the Implementation Plan.*
2. *The NIH Corporate Role in the Implementation Plan.*
3. *Science Programs will be the Focus of NIH Budget Presentations.*
4. *Commitment to Scientifically Meritorious Investigator-Initiated Research.*
5. *Balance/Diversity of the NIH Research Portfolio.*
6. *Adherence to the Principles of Cost Management.*

■ **Office of Technology Assessment. *Federally Funded Research: Decisions for a Decade*. Washington, D.C.: U.S. Government Printing Office, 1992.**

In December 1989, the House Committee on Science, Space, and Technology requested that OTA assist it in understanding the state of the federally funded research system—its goals, research choices, policies, and outcomes—and the challenges that it will face in the 1990s.

Today, because the scientific community has the capability to undertake far more research than the Federal Government supports, policymakers and sponsors of research must continuously choose between competing "goods."

Given the extraordinary strength of the U.S. research system and the character of scientific research, there will always be more opportunities than can be funded, more researchers competing than can be sustained, and more institutions seeking to expand than the prime sponsor—the Federal Government—can fund. The objective, then, is to ensure that the best research continues to be funded, that a full portfolio of research is maintained, and that there is a sufficient research work force of the highest caliber to do the job.

The distribution of Federal research and development (R&D) funds has long been a contentious issue—both in Congress and in the scientific community. . . if these funds are aggregated by the State of the recipient institution or laboratory, then five States received 53 percent of the R&D funds in fiscal year 1990.

At the institutional level, 10 universities receive 25 percent of the Federal research funding, and only 30 universities account for 50 percent. Funding is concentrated in 100 research universities in 38 States.

These data on the distribution of resources bear a critical message: research capabilities—institutions and people—take time to grow. It is not simply a matter of "they who have, get." The reputation, talent, and infrastructure of research universities attract researchers and graduate students. Some universities become assets not only in the production of fundamental knowledge, but also in bridging science and technology to other goals such as State and regional economic development.

Measures of distress and conflicts over resource allocation within the scientific community do not address whether the Nation needs more science. Other problems in the Federal research system do not derive from, but are exacerbated by, such stress. They include sparse participation by women and ethnic minorities in science, indications that other nations are better able to capitalize on the results of U.S. research than American industry, and management problems that have plagued many Federal research agencies.

In the 1990s the Federal research system will face many challenges. OTA has organized them here under four interrelated issues: 1) setting priorities for the support of research; 2) understanding research expenditures; 3) adapting education and human resources to meet the changing needs of the research work force; and 4) refining data collection, analysis, and interpretation to improve Federal decisionmaking.

■ **Pardes H. Assessing the past and planning the future to ensure support for biomedical research.** *Academic Medicine.* **1991;66: 582-584.**

Reprinted with permission of *Academic Medicine* (formerly the *Journal of Medical Education*).

The author notes the current extraordinary excitement and opportunity in biomedical research that, oddly, exist within a context of economic constraint for researchers. Also, there is much negative publicity about biomedical science that threatens efforts to obtain adequate funding and responsible handling of science policy in an era where there is relatively little money available for research. The author reviews past instances of damaging public disunity and squabbles by groups in the biomedical research community and then proposes various policy guidelines and strategies to best ensure adequate research funding in the future. For such policies and guidelines to be effective, he stresses the necessity of efforts to heal the past divisions within the biomedical research community and to present a united position that is clear and understandable to Congress and others.

Should the average duration of grants be reduced from the current average of 4.3 years? I believe a slight decrease would not unduly traumatize the scientific community, but an excessive reduction would exacerbate the problem of excessive time and effort spent in grant writing and grant evaluation.

Should downward negotiations be eliminated? Probably yes, but the process may have to be phased out rather than abruptly ended. Downward negotiations contribute to the growing uncertainty and tension in the scientific community.

To tamper with indirect costs plays havoc with the ability of many of the strongest research universities to do science. Also, to introduce cost as a criterion when assessing scientific projects is dangerous.

In essence, research is in the political arena, and scientists have to learn to assert in that arena. We are competing for funds with many other societal programs. We believe increased support of our programs is in the public's best interest. Given that fact, we must do the work needed to justify our claims and secure support.

■ Pavitt K. What makes basic research economically useful? *Research Policy.* 1991;20:109-119.

Reprinted with permisison of Elsevier Science Publishers B.V.

Economic analysis has helped us understand the strong economic dimension in the explosive growth of science, and (more recently) the reasons for continuing public subsidies. However, the growing domination of the "market failure" approach has led to the analytical neglect of two major questions for policy-makers. How does science contribute to technology? Are the technological benefits from science increasingly becoming international?

On the former, too much attention has been devoted to the relatively narrow range of scientific fields producing knowledge with direct technological applications, and too little to the much broader range of fields, the skills of which contribute to most technologies. On the latter, national systems of science and of technology remain closely coupled in most major countries, in spite of the technological activities of large multinational firms.

Empirical research is needed on concentration, scale and efficiency in the performance of basic research, where techniques and insights from the applied economics of industrial R&D are of considerable relevance. There is no convincing evidence so far of unexploited economies of scale in basic research.

This evidence shows that many policies for greater "selectivity and concentration" in basic research have been misconceived. Economists and other social scientists could help by formulating more persuasive justifications for public subsidy for basic research, and by making more realistic assumptions about the nature of science and technology.

■ **President's Council of Advisors on Science and Technology.** *Renewing the Promise: Research-Intensive Universities and the Nation.* **Washington, D.C.: United States Government Printing Office, 1992.**

The human and intellectual capital generated by U.S. colleges and universities over the past four decades has been the basis for a vast array of accomplishments that have touched the lives of all Americans.

Those accomplishments notwithstanding, the relationship between the American public and institutions of higher learning is showing serious signs of stress. This partnership of over one hundred and fifty research-intensive universities and the federal government has grown to be a research and educational enterprise of enormous size, scope, and complexity. Despite their success, or perhaps in part because of the ever increasing expectations derived from that success, universities are losing public confidence.

In reviewing the health of the nation's research-intensive universities and their relationship with the federal government, PCAST has focused on six main areas:
- the implications of a limited resource environment;
- the fundamental importance of teaching activities at research-intensive universities;
- the erosion of public trust and confidence in our universities;
- federal investment in university-based research;
- interactions between universities and industry;
- and the identification and development of exceptional talent for science and technology.

So that research-intensive universities may continue to function productively in an environment of limited resources, PCAST urges them to:

adopt more highly selective strategies based on a realistic appraisal of the future availability of resources and a commitment to meet world-class standards in all programs that are undertaken.

Such strategies will require universities to:

- eliminate or downsize some departments and specialties;
- collaborate with other academic, industrial, and governmental institutions;
- build facilities or programs only where there are strong long-term prospects of sustaining them; and
- develop permanent institutional mechanisms for strategic planning . . . .

Universities should reemphasize teaching in all its aspects, both inside and outside the classroom. In doing so, many institutions will have to curtail some of their research activities.

PCAST recommends that universities strengthen their educational functions by:

- increasing direct senior faculty involvement in teaching . . . ;
- balancing the contributions of teaching . . . with those of research and public service in evaluating and rewarding faculty;
- placing less reliance on graduate teaching assistants . . . ;
- increasing the involvement of undergraduates in hands-on frontier research; . . .

. . . the university community and its patrons, including federal agencies, must act in ways designed to preserve the core values that underlie the scientific and educational enterprise—free and creative pursuit of ideas and synergism between research and teaching.

. . . PCAST makes specific recommendations to federal agencies. . . . They address: full federal reimbursement of all legitimate indirect costs; the growing obsolescence of the physical infrastructure for university-based research; improvements in the administration of federal research support to universities; and reexamination of the role of federal laboratories.

Some of the cultural differences that have long surrounded industrial research and university research have had the unfortunate effect of unnecessarily inhibiting the most effective interaction between industry and universities.

. . . PCAST recommends that:

- universities and industry together, through a wide range of concerted actions, should exchange scientists and engineers at all levels—especially their very best—between the two sectors for substantial periods of time and repeatedly throughout their careers.

Stronger public policies must be designed to identify scientifically gifted persons at an early age and to help them develop their talents to the fullest, no matter what their circumstances.

■ Senker J. Evaluating the funding of strategic science: some lessons from British experience. *Research Policy.* 1991;20:29-43.

Reprinted with permission of Elsevier Science Publishers B.V.

Considerable emphasis is currently being placed on funding strategic research in universities. This paper presents the background to the development of this policy and then discusses the response of the Science and Engineering Research Council (SERC). In particular it focuses on the SERC's Directorate programmes for fostering strategic research, and assesses some outcomes from this approach. An evaluation of the Biotechnology Directorate provides the main basis for the paper, but evaluations of other Directorates are also drawn on.

The two central questions discussed are the success of Directorates at building up the science base and their effectiveness at promoting technology transfer to industry. The paper concludes that Directorate programmes have achieved a great measure of success in meeting these objectives, but in so doing have raised further questions, including how large a proportion of funds should be allocated to strategic as opposed to "blue sky" research.

. . . perhaps most crucial to the vitality of basic science, there is the requirement to evaluate regularly the continuing need and overall level of funding for strategic research. Initiatives to promote strategic research in universities may be important during specific periods of time, but institutional inertia must be overcome in order to ensure that when new technologies reach maturity the balance shifts back towards basic science once again.

■ Sherman JF. Shaping national science policy: some lessons learned. *Academic Medicine.* 1991;66:66-70.

Reprinted with permission of *Academic Medicine* (formerly the *Journal of Medical Education*).

Thirty-five years of experience have taught several lessons about shaping science policy. Derived from these lessons are four premises that deserve individual and collective thought: (1) The partnership in U.S. society between health and science interests is fundamentally important; (2) Scientific merit must be the paramount basis for allocating whatever research funds are available; (3) Better data and their careful analysis are vital to the decision-making processes; and (4) More than ever we must have a clear, concise, vigorous, and repeated enunciation of the principles that are essential for a national biomedical research program to flourish. The fourth premise is expressed succinctly in the 11 principles outlined in the 1983 AAMC monograph "Preserving America's Preeminence in Medical Research," which places important responsibilities for the collective success of the

U.S. research program on all of the various components of society. Three important factors favor efforts to shape a useful, successful science policy: a public that places improvements in health high on every priority list, a rapidly expanding body of invaluable knowledge, and a sizable investment of tax-derived funds, now totalling over $7.5 billion per year.

■ **Tauber AI, Sarkar S. The Human Genome Project: has blind reductionism gone too far?** *Perspectives in Biology and Medicine.* **1992;35:220-235.**

The Human Genome Project (HGP) is now well under way.

The purpose of this article is, first, to evaluate critically the scientific merit of the project; second, to very briefly suggest that the project is the culmination of a research program within biology that, for 2 centuries, has been fundamentally reductionist; and, third, to conclude that the doubts raised about the scientific merits of the project may well illustrate the limitations of such reductionist approaches in biology (and, perhaps even more strongly, in medicine) at present.

The HGP is the ultimate product of an extreme reductionist vision of biology that has held that *to understand better one need only to go smaller.* Reductionism in molecular biology constitutes a research program that attempts to explain and understand biological systems completely in terms of the physical interactions of their parts. From that point of view, it is natural to assume that fundamental understanding of biology comes only from the level of DNA, the alleged blueprint for living systems.

This article has emphasized the scientific shortcomings of the HGP. It is important to note, as many have pointed out, that the original design of the HGP has been extensively modified as a result of criticism and concerns over the scientific legitimacy of its initial goals. The only consensus that has survived is a limited acquiescence to the idea of mapping. That consensus has not been challenged here. Rather, the criticisms offered are of the original and ultimate aims of the HGP: namely, blind sequencing.

In conclusion, it is important to reemphasize that biological systems are complex, largely hierarchically organized, interacting systems; to understand them, the most critical investigation is that of the function of units at each level of organization. This has largely been the purpose of biological research; in even as reductionist a science as molecular biology, few would argue with Davis: "Our fundamental goal is to understand the human genome and its products, and not to sequence the genome because it is there." After the initial reductionist euphoria of the 1950s and early 1960s, molecular biology has often paid attention to such problems in spite of generally being reductionist: hence the interest in studies of molecular evolution, of development at the molecular level, and of molecular mechanisms that mediate the neural or immunological systems. But these, like the other examples mentioned above, are problems independently known to be of biological importance. In many of these areas, progress has been unexpectedly slow, but perhaps the lesson to be learned is not the desirability of more reduction but less—the lack of progress may well be due to the limits of blind reductionism itself. If these considerations have any merit, the blind sequencing of the HGP is an unfortunate step backward.

■ **Yager T, Nickerson D, Hood L. The Human Genome Project: creating an infrastructure for biology and medicine.** *Trends in Biochemical Sciences.* **1991;16:454-461.**

Reprinted with permission of Elsevier Trends Journals.

The Human Genome Project (HGP) is an international effort to map and sequence the human genome. It combines skills from diverse fields of biological and technological research, thus establishing deeper interactions between scientific disciplines. The combination of these skills should stimulate many advances in both pure and applied fields of research and give rise to new, interdisciplinary training programs. Some critics say that the HGP will damage biomedical research; however, we argue that it will bring new funds to the field and create a large ripple effect by providing new research opportunities through its discoveries.

The HGP will have several long-term positive effects on science and society. (1) It will foster a deeper interaction between biology, medicine and other academic disciplines. (2) The technology for genome mapping, sequencing and analysis will be pushed to a much higher level. (3) As the database of genetic, physical and sequence maps becomes generally accessible, there will be a dramatic effect on the practice of biology. (4) Access to a database of genetic, physical and sequence maps will also fundamentally change the practice of clinical medicine.

Of course, the HGP also has long-term implications that defy a simple analysis of costs and benefits. There is, for example, a potential for misuse of information by groups in society, particularly in the realm of genetic diagnosis. We do not presume to answer critics who raise profound questions in the fields of ethics, law and sociology. We note, however, that the HGP is not unique in this respect, since many scientific revolutions have ultimately been catalysts of social change.

Neil S. Cherniack

I t is reasonable to believe that public support for biomedical research is based on the expectation that research leads to improved health and not just to new knowledge. This mission has been perhaps clearer to the physician than to the non-physician scientist. While the biomedical research program has been enormously successful in generating new knowledge and has made the United States the world leader in biomedical research, it has been less obviously successful in improving health. It is this relative lack of success in its applied mission that has placed public financing of biomedical research at risk and endangers the ability to capitalize on discoveries in basic research.

While biomedical research has not caused the problems in health care the U.S. is experiencing (although to some it may have), it clearly has been less attentive to these problems than it might or should have been. The fundamental problem in biomedical research now is how best to achieve the same success in applied research as it has in basic research, without interfering with the enormous capabilities that have been developed to advance basic research. The answer may be that this is impossible unless there is a serious rethinking of how we conduct research.

The major issues in biomedical research can be expressed as follows:

How do we maintain a balanced list of priorities that allows research grants to be funded, attracts and trains research investigators, and allows for adequate research equipment and facilities? Will "Big Science" interfere with our ability to carry out research which traditionally has taken place in the "Small Science" mode? Do we need a master plan to achieve our research goals?

Finally, although not mentioned in the articles selected, there is the issue of how the academic health center and physicians should participate in the research effort.

Successful research requires adequate facilities, accurate instruments, and talented and trained investigators. Brilliant ideas are important, but they are simply not enough. We all know stories of chance conversations producing the ideas that lead to major advances in biological sciences and in medicine. We often tend to forget the immense resources that are required to allow great ideas to reach fruition. It is important to remember that the chance discussions in which these ideas may arise occur in fertile settings in which there were already sizeable numbers of investigators, laboratories, technicians, and equipment.

Although individual initiative, as exemplified in RO-1 funded research, remains a vital element in biomedical research, research is no longer a cottage industry. Cutting edge research takes place ever more often where there are large groups of scientists working in related areas, communicating with each other effectively and working together cooperatively. In a sense, Big Science (though not in the NASA sense) has been here for many years. It seems likely that it is here to stay and will be increasingly important as the complexity and cost of instrumentation increase and the ability to generate scientific knowledge accelerates.

This does not necessarily mean that biomedical research will ultimately be concentrated in a few centers. The increased ability to exchange information (e.g., words, numbers, and pictures) rapidly and accurately should make it possible for networks of small groups of investigators who are miles apart to work together effectively on basic research projects. Clinical trials of drugs and the assessment of health outcomes obviously require this network approach. Big Science networking, however, requires much greater planning than has heretofore been the case both at the regional and central levels. Whether or not we agree with the details of the NIH strategic plan, we should commend the efforts to develop such a plan.

Research has, as has health care, become increasingly expensive. But biomedical research dollars, particularly from governmental agencies, have become more limited. Commercial sources (e.g., pharmaceutical companies, biotechnology corporations, even insurance companies) have always contributed to research. It seems that the importance of this support will become greater. Clearly we will need to protect academic interests in an environment where biomedical research has as one of its goals not only the health of the people but also the health of the economy. Perhaps this can be accomplished by partnerships between the university and commercial entities which also involve either community agencies and voluntary health organizations or the organizations that exist in many states to encourage industrial growth and create jobs.

The academic health center must and should continue to play a very significant role in biomedical research. This institution is already organized to carry out research at both the very basic and at the quite applied levels. In addition, the academic health center is able to construct the bridges between basic and applied research. These bridges are essential if the relevance of basic research is to be appreciated, its potential in health care realized, and basic scientists are to become familiar with the contribution they can make to solving major health problems.

How important is the physician to the research effort? Clearly the physician is an essential member of research endeavors that deal with humans, particularly studies to test the efficacy of new diagnostic procedures and novel therapeutic regimens.

We also need physicians to engage in basic research even if merely to help form some of the connecting links between the laboratory bench and the patient. However, I suspect that the number of physicians engaged in bench research will decrease as more and more demands are placed on medical schools to turn out practitioners, particularly primary care doctors.

Perhaps we need a new kind of primary care physician. Research in primary care specialties has focused on population-based studies. Primary care physicians typically do not engage in bench research, but there is no reason why they could not. One might even make the case that MD-PhD programs should attempt to direct their students to primary care because a broad-based clinical expertise would be of much greater value to a bench researcher than would highly specialized clinical information. In the past, research was based on the study of the body's organs. It seemed natural therefore that the cardiologist would lead research projects designed to answer questions in heart disease. However, present-day research is based in cell and molecular biology and not necessarily directed to specific organ problems.

Bench research has become increasingly a full-time occupation. It could be argued that just as other healthcare personnel are replacing physicians in some of their clinical roles, a new kind of person may extend or replace the physician in research. We ought to consider the possibility of developing a new kind of post-graduate program for PhDs which allows them to gain experience with patients and provides insights into clinical problems. We may also want to develop new kinds of residency programs for the MD-PhD students that allow them to continue bench research while they are being trained clinically.

It is clear that we need to rethink the organization of research recognizing that the academic health center's role in the research enterprise remains crucial. Academic health centers must create new linkages with each other, with industry, and with the community. The academic health center must also train new kinds of research personnel who can bridge basic and applied science interests and apply the new ideas developed by the basic scientists to human health problems.

CHAPTER IV

Biotechnology, Biomedical Research, and Global Competition

ABSTRACTS AND EXCERPTS

■ **Burton DF. A new model for U.S. innovation.** *Issues in Science and Technology.* **1992;8:52-59.**

The United States will not be able to ensure technological leadership simply by focusing more R&D on specific areas; it must reassess its entire approach to innovation. Many of the assumptions underlying the U.S. innovation system are out of touch with the demands of today's international marketplace, and the policies based on them must be redirected.

The U.S. government has a long tradition of funding national technology initiatives, from the Manhattan Project to the Human Genome Initiative. . . . The key policy question is whether the government adequately takes into account competitiveness concerns in making these funding decisions. There is a growing consensus among industry leaders that it does not.

The basic problem is that the traditional model treats industrial technology as an incidental dividend of government R&D missions, rather than as the primary objective.

To sustain a competitive edge in the twenty-first century, we must understand the false assumptions that underlie the traditional model, replace them with relevant assumptions that are true to the international marketplace, and establish a set of new, vital, and effective policies that will foster a dynamic alliance between government and industry.

The nation will need new kinds of innovation policies in the future. They can be divided into five areas: involving the private sector in setting new national R&D priorities; promoting technology diffusion; strengthening the U.S. technology infrastructure; improving U.S. manufacturing process technology; and tracking technology and global markets.

■ **Davis EB, Weiner JL, Farber NJ, Boyer EG, Robinson EJ. Watching the biotech window of opportunity.** *J of Amer Health Policy.* **1992;2:52-55.**

Reprinted with permission of Faulkner & Gray, Inc.

. . . the research reported on in this article focuses on an assessment of attitudes of future management and medical leaders in the biotechnology industry in an effort to better understand the dynamics of decision making and management systems aimed at biotechnology product development. The study population in this research included MBA and medical students comparing and contrasting the two populations' attitudes with regard to key process issues facing the biotechnology field.

Specific issues examined included: human biological materials (human tissues/organs) as commodities, legislation and policy governing the biotechnology industry, and economic transactions associated with the acquisition and distribution of human biological materials.

Our findings suggest that, as the biotechnology industry grows, human biological materials will continue to be perceived as valuable commodities. In addition, despite the call for a more organized system to monitor and regulate the acquisition and distribution of human tissues/organs, government involvement is not seen as a highly desirable characteristic for infrastructure development.

The management attitudes reflected in this research would point toward the development of an industry in which organizational strategy would be built upon competitive market acquisition of human biological materials through pricing; product innovation through harvester revenue sharing contract arrangements; exclusion of supplier benefits from commercial product margins; and little governmental intervention and regulation.

■ **Office of Technology Assessment.** *Biotechnology in a global economy.* **Washington, D.C.: Office of Technology Assessment, 1992.**

Biotechnology—both as a scientific art and commercial entity—is less than 20 years old. In that short period of time, however, it has revolutionized the way scientists view living matter and has resulted in research and development (R&D) that may lead to commercialization of products that can dramatically improve human and animal health, the food supply, and the quality of the environment. Developed primarily in U.S. laboratories, many applications of biotechnology are now viewed by companies and governments throughout the world as essential for economic growth in several different, seemingly disparate industries.

This report describes the increasing international use of commercial biotechnology in industrialized and newly industrializing countries (NICs) and the ways governments promote and regulate the uses of biotechnology.

U.S. competitiveness in the global commercialization of biotechnology has come to the attention of Congress for three reasons. First, the U.S. Government indirectly supports industrial applications of biotechnology by funding basic research in a wide range of relevant disciplines. Second, Federal agencies have the authority to regulate the commercial development of biotechnology. Third, international economic competitiveness in various technologies, including biotechnology, has emerged as a key bipartisan concern.

In all three areas, Congress plays a direct role. Through its annual appropriations to Federal agencies, it increases or decreases the level of research and regulatory oversight. Through its authorization powers, Congress can create programs and set priorities for Federal agencies. Through oversight of agencies' conduct of research and regulatory programs, Congress can express its enthusiasm and concern.

Seven policy issues relevant to U.S. competitiveness in biotechnology were identified during the course of this study:

- Federal funding for biotechnology research,
- targeting biotechnology development,
- developing regulations,
- coordinating Federal agencies,
- protecting intellectual property,
- improving industry-university relationships, and
- structuring coherent tax policies.

■ **Vaughan C, Smith BL, Porter RJ. U.S. biomedical science and technology.** *Knowledge: Creation, Diffusion, Utilization.* **1992; 14:91-109.**

. . . we examine the *impact* of this shift in expectations on medicine and medical research, the financial impact of health research, and most especially, the competitive implication of the health care revolution in the United States. The aim is to assess how the United States can maintain a continuous improvement in health care with advanced technologies and sustain its position as world leader in research and development of those technologies.

The extraordinary growth of the medical industry has been paradoxical in its effect . . . for medical technology is not only a powerful and important sector of the economy but also a potential drain on the GNP.

Payments from the federal government account for a sizable fraction of what consumers expend for health care, hence prompting the critics of what is often called the "health-industrial complex" to complain that public expenditures, and not market forces, produce the dynamic growth of the medical technology and pharmaceutical industries.

As the nation seeks to control medical costs, measures that reduce access to some medical treatments will evoke an opposing political pressure to spend the money necessary to provide the medical care that people expect. There is little reason to expect health care costs to decrease markedly despite strenuous cost-containment efforts.

The billions in products that are currently produced in the United States to satisfy U.S. demand could as easily be produced in other industrialized nations. If one country does not produce them, others likely will do so. The trade deficit could thus be exacerbated if the United States were to lose its technological edge in medical devices and biomedicine. *Such a situation would give the United States the worst of both worlds: escalating health care costs and dependence on foreign sources of supply.*

Among the factors that potentially constrain the U.S. biomedical industry, the failure to invest sufficiently in research and development (R&D) is a major concern.

Political efforts to control prices also can make some areas of research and development appear unprofitable.

Even more important, perhaps, are tax policies and the cost of capital that affect the pace of innovation in the drug industry.

In addition to financial considerations, government regulations can be a constraint on any industry. Because people's health is potentially at risk, the biomedical industry will inevitably be strongly regulated. . . . the rising cost of medical care is likely to invite more economic controls.

All of the aforementioned constraints are external to the biomedical business or research center, but there are also constraining factors that can exist inside organizations. Ultimately, these internal variables may be the most important determinants of the future health of the whole industry. An overly conservative approach to new projects among industrial managers can stifle creativity and block new ventures. A conservative attitude on the part of university administrators can similarly discourage faculty interaction with industry.

For the U.S. biomedical industry to maintain its lead it must be sensitive to the new dynamics of biomedical product development, recognizing that (1) the "milking" of current products without investment in the future is suicidal; (2) no lead can be considered comfortable with the dynamic technology of today's highly competitive environment; (3) the trend toward increasing research investment by all companies and increasing capital costs of research is here to stay; (4) protectionism is not the wave of the future and is a counterproductive means to solve the problems of industrial indolence; and (5) risks in new fields of research are unavoidable. Special attention must be given to developments in the new biotechnology, which will soon be a dominant force in biomedical research, technological development, and product sales.

COMMENTARY
Leslie S. Cutler

The United States is the acknowledged world leader in biotechnology research and the biotechnology industry. Biotechnology and biomedical research are indeed significant components in America's industrial portfolio that can help our nation to compete effectively in the evolving global economy.

One of the great competitive strengths of the United States has been our highly effective system of research and development. For example, this is the system that created most of the products which are the heart of the world's consumer electronics industry: the color television, the phonograph, both the audio and video tape recorders, the telephone, and the integrated circuit. Today, however, American industry builds only a fraction of the electronics products purchased in this and other countries. It is said that the United States in no longer competitive in many industrial arenas such as the consumer electronics, automotive, and the steel industries. At the moment, that is not the case in the areas of biotechnology and biomedical research.

How can we avoid the mistakes that were made in these other industries and ensure that we capitalize on our strengths in biotechnology and biomedical research? How can we leverage our world leadership in biotechnology to help our national economy and to enhance our position in the global marketplace?

It is clear that our nation's biotechnology research and development capabilities are strong. That strength comes from a stable and secure university system of basic research that has its foundations in our nation's research universities. This academic research base is enhanced by a strong industrial (pharmaceutical and biotechnology) commitment to research and development. We must continue to support and nurture basic research at our nation's universities and in industry. We must ensure the provision of a modern, state-of-the-art research infrastructure that supports this effort. It is this basic research that provides the bulk of the "raw material" from which new, marketable products can be developed. Many of the findings of today's basic molecular biologic research often lead, quite directly, to marketable products. In fact, these results can become the products or the tools for manufacturing these products. Thus, cloning the gene for a hormone such as insulin yields both the product and the basic means for generating commercial quantities of the hormone.

Quite unexpectedly, in this new era of science, basic research and applied research have grown so close they are often inseparable. Thus, the loss of basic science research could represent the loss of the products as well as the means for their production. Very rapidly, the country could lose its advantage in this highly competitive global marketplace that offers substantial potential for growth and expansion.

Currently, nearly 70 percent of all of the activity in biotechnology is focused on developing therapeutic or diagnostic products for human health care. However, the nation's biotechnological advantage transcends the biomedical field. Indeed, it opens new opportunities in a wide variety of markets. The molecular biologic and other tools of the biotechnology industry have the potential to create new products which can impact many other arenas. The impact of biotechnology in the fields of agriculture (e.g., fast-growing, high-yield, disease-resistant crops and improved livestock) and marine science (e.g., aquaculture as a food resource, and new pharmaceuticals) is already apparent. Less obvious, perhaps, is the potential to use biotechnologically altered or created farm and marine animals as renewable, nonpolluting "biologic factories." Other creative opportunities await discovery by clever scientists exploiting these evolving technologies.

Often overlooked is the potential impact these biotechnologies can have as a source for new products and processes in a diverse array of markets not normally associated with biological systems. For example, the technology is showing great promise in the areas of environmental protection and cleanup. This is a market that will have increasing importance in the future as the world is faced with developing new, cost-effective ways to protect and clean the environment. Biotechnology has been emerging as a method for the synthesis and commercial production of alternative fuels that will help to conserve existing fossil fuels while offering the potential for higher energy efficiency and less environmental pollution. The application of biotechnology could lead to new approaches to processing chemical and petrochemical products. The use of biologic systems to synthesize commercially valuable membranes which could serve as filters in various filtration or concentration systems is another potential market application. Biologically engineered systems are being developed to serve as biosensing or bioprocessing units to assist in a variety of manufacturing and quality control systems. Finally, the coupling of biotechnology with the new nanotechnology offers potentials for future products and manufacturing opportunities yet to be discovered.

We must invest in and protect these new technologies, as they represent the competitive advantage the country will need to remain strong in the new and diversifying global economy. We cannot sustain our economy by being a service nation or by being a nation that invents new products and processes that other countries ultimately manufacture. We must invest in both the science and the application of this science for commercial use.

Higher education, especially research universities, cannot flourish if the country does not survive economically. It is in the best interest of all segments of the society for universities, government, and industry to form partnerships which leverage and protect our current technological edge in the biotechnology arena to build products and manufacturing capabilities that can help sustain the nation's economic future in the evolving global economy.

COMMENTARY

Cynthia Maurer-Sutton and William N. Kelley

"Biotech" spans the entire gamut from fundamental research in academe, to the application of this research for commercial use in the biotech industry, to pharmaceutical companies that often are the entities that bring biotechnology through commercialization and make it available to the public.

The United States has led the world in biotech due to a strong research base, the industrial capacity to translate basic research into products, and the ability to finance research ideas. Biotech will likely be the principal scientific driving force behind the discovery of new drugs and therapies in the next century. This enterprise is therefore important to our nation, which currently has the technological and therefore the economic leadership in this field. In 1989, biomedicine resulted in a trade surplus of $2.3 billion for the United States. It is interesting to note that a large number of Japanese scholars have participated in research training programs in the U.S. to try to export this expertise to their home country. It is clear that if American companies do not produce in the biomedical area, others will do so. If the United States loses this technological edge, we could have the worst of both worlds: escalating healthcare costs and American companies that fear delays in recouping their development costs and decide not to compete. Thus the American people would become dependent on foreign companies.

Competitiveness and the global commercialization of biotech have come to the attention of the U.S. Congress, because the government indirectly supports industrial applications of biotech by funding basic research primarily in universities. In addition, since the United States is the world leader in biotechnology, an area that contributes significantly to our economy, it has become a major area of focus of international economic competitiveness.

In order to understand how to enhance and help facilitate the biotech area, it is important to understand the significant number of challenges facing the field today: product development moved slower than expected; tightened venture-capital financing because expected returns on investments have not materialized; the significant amount of financing that is required to bridge the gap between the basic research and the marketable product. (As much as $5-10 billion may still be needed to develop over 100 biotech products currently in clinical trials.)

U.S. firms are also disadvantaged when it comes to acquisitions due to accounting practices that limit the deduction of their research and development expenses in the year expended; the higher costs of capital facing U.S. firms relative to foreign firms; and an insufficient supply of well-trained, basic scientists and clinical investigators needed in academe and industry.

There are many countries that have already developed governmental industrial policies that promote biotech due to its importance to the country's future development (e.g., Japan, Korea). Based on the factors noted above, it is evident that the U.S. needs to develop an academic-industrial policy that supports the development of biotech, and thus enhances the competitiveness of America in this key area. The policy might include the following elements:

1. Funding of Biomedical Research

   The funding of biomedical research must be increased with the well-established process of peer review used to allocate these funds, thus ensuring that the most meritorious and sound basic and clinical research is identified.

   One of the primary research goals is to improve the health of people. Industry, on the other hand, is a critical catalyst for bringing fundamental research advances to market. Both academe and industry are key and must be supported if we are to continue our global success. Lobbying groups must not become part of the allocation process. If decisions about this country's research are based on efforts of the commercial sector in a political setting rather than the expertise that comes with scientific peer review, Congress will be overwhelmed by lobbyists and advocacy groups urging narrow agendas. America's ability to understand and fight the myriad diseases and disabilities we face will be engulfed in a quagmire.

2. Recognize biotech as a key area for growth and increase international presence

We need to recognize the importance of biotech to the health of the U.S. economy, and determine how we are performing relative to the rest of the world. We need to begin to track technology in global markets and to increase our foreign presence. Burton notes, "The United States maintains 50,000 troops in Japan, but only five commercial officers. By contrast, the Japan External Trade Organization, which gathers commercial information and explores market opportunities, has several hundred officers in New York City alone (and obviously no troops)."

3. Enhance effectiveness of federal agencies

The Food and Drug Administration (FDA) has done a good job in facilitating the review process when it has identified new unique fields, such as gene therapy. It is recommended that the FDA and other agencies review their approval processes to determine if revisions can be made to appropriately facilitate the transfer of biotechnology even further.

The Recombinant DNA Advisory Committee (RAC) of the NIH has recently abolished its human gene therapy subcommittee in order to facilitate program review. On the other hand, the pipeline of new biological products for approval by the FDA remains very long.

4. Protection of intellectual property

The protection of intellectual property is a very important factor when addressing a country's competitiveness in such new fields as biomedicine. There are a number of elements that affect competitiveness when considering the protection of intellectual property. First, there is a serious backlog at the Patent and Trademark Offices because there are uncertainties regarding what constitutes patentable subject matter. Second, the procedural option of an accelerated examination is rarely used for biotech applications. Therefore the length of time for review is considerable. In addition, as this complex field continues to evolve at such a rapid pace, the ability of inventors to understand and to easily meet the procedural requirements of various patent offices will probably become an important factor.

5. Enhancing the technology transfer of biomedicine

Since most of the biomedicine is being developed in academe and then transferred into industry, it is important to look at how we can facilitate this transfer of technology. Below are recommendations to help in this transfer:

- Support of clinical investigators

  The explosion of new knowledge in biomedicine will create the need for more expertise, particularly fully trained physicians to transform these discoveries into cost-effective treatments for human disease. However, at this time there are many factors discouraging the brightest and best individuals from pursuing this career path. In order to make this field more attractive to the best candidates, we need to look at developing policies that address critical issues that include: relief of medical school debt; financial support during residency training; research training and appropriate fellowships; and initial research awards for young faculty.[1]

- Support appropriate university-industry relationships

  There have been documented benefits that support the continuation and further development of university-industry relationships. Legislation that restricts the ability of publicly funded researchers to collaborate with industry could discourage the entrepreneurial initiative of scientists and possibly limit the value of their research. Therefore, we need to review how to encourage appropriate university-industry relationships that both address and avoid potential conflict of interest issues.

- Development of incubator facilities and funding sources for start-ups

  The development of incubator facilities and the identification of funding sources for biotech companies are important to the technology transfer process. Most biomedicine developed in academe is too embryonic to commercialize; it must be further developed. However, the cost is prohibitive, and it does not support the mission of academe to perform all of such research in its laboratories. Therefore, true incubator space, which is ideally structured for the development of this emerging technology, must be developed. This development also has its costs. As the venture capital financing market has tightened, we must consider how the start-ups can identify funding sources.

6. Structure appropriate tax policies

In analyzing how to support the development of the biotech area, the tax policies with regard to the research and development tax credit and the amortization of goodwill should be reviewed to determine if they support the development of biomedicine and the global competitiveness of U.S. industry that is trying to commercialize this technology. Some believe that the research and development tax credit should be refundable rather than being carried forward to be used against future earnings because industry (especially start-ups) requires cash flow now, not sometime in the future. In addition, we should review the inability of U.S. firms to amortize goodwill for tax purposes as quickly as foreign firms.

7. Alliance for Health Research

The Institute of Medicine recently recommended the formation of an alliance among the Executive Branch, Congress, industry, foundations, and academe for health research, calling it paramount to this nation's ability to find both the will and the way to address our clinical research needs and the translation of fundamental research into high quality, cost-effective health care. The recommended first step is the creation of a Federal Task Force, to be coordinated by the President's Office of Science and Technology Policy, to convene the key federal agencies and other stakeholders, such as academic medicine and the pharmaceutical, biotechnology, and insurance companies. The purpose of the task force would be to highlight and promote the importance of clinical research to the future health and welfare of the American people and the nation's economic competitiveness as well as to analyze steps that can be undertaken to enhance clinical research and to lay the foundation for future collaborative efforts through an Alliance for Health Research.[2]

Biomedical research and the transfer of this technology to the market are extremely important to the health and welfare of the American people and to our nation's global competitiveness. It is important for the government to define an industrial policy that supports the continued development of this complex area, which is evolving at an exponential pace. This policy must recognize the contributions of academe and industry in the development and commercialization of the technology, and identify policies that provide incentives and appropriately support this development.

COMMENTARY

Manuel Tzagournis

Strong basic science has placed the United States in a leadership position in biotechnology and biomedical research. A successful partnership exists between government and research universities with their academic health centers. That system is responsible for producing scientific innovations that impact dramatically on multiple aspects of our lives. Add to that an entrepreneurial private industry that provides generous venture capital along with expertise, and one finds a formidable competitive force in the world.

Although the United States is the undisputed leader in biotechnology and biomedical discovery, global economic competition is keen. Scientific discovery of new technology does not suffice to maintain a leadership position. Witness the losses to other countries in recent times that we experienced in other high technology areas such as computer memory chips. Technology transfer and application to commercial uses are expertly accomplished by countries such as Japan and Germany. These countries excel in making incremental improvements in products and in developing efficient quality manufacturing systems. It is likely that major old-fashioned wars will be displaced by global economic wars. Biotechnology and biomedical research will be important battle grounds in those wars.

How should we prepare for such competition in the global economy? Burton's article suggests several policy directions that are quite reasonable in my view. The federal government should take competitiveness into account in making policy or funding decisions while enthusiastically continuing to support basic research. New strategies should be directed toward improving the technology infrastructure and manufacturing processes. If we ignore these, we are destined to repeat some of the mistakes that occurred in other areas of innovations. As pointed out in the article, "Biotechnology in a Global Economy," there are two prerequisites for a nation to fully compete in this arena: (1) a strong research base and (2) the industrial capacity to convert the research into desired products.

It is encouraging that U.S. Commerce Secretary Ron Brown has repeated President Clinton's campaign pledge to invest in "technologies that could prove critical to economic growth." Equally important is a commitment to appropriate polices that encourage every step of biotechnology from discovery of new knowledge to its application in biological pharmaceuticals, agriculture, human health, or the environment. In addition to initiatives to fund basic research and to develop the research infrastructure, the federal agencies involved in biotechnology should focus on achieving additional goals, namely, emphasis on interdisciplinary research and an increase in training programs.

From the perspective of an academician in a large public university, it is important to educate policymakers and to reach the public. The state of Ohio, for example, has a relatively balanced economy comprising manufacturing, agriculture, and services that would benefit greatly from biotechnology and biomedical research. The formation of a biotechnology center at The Ohio State University serves the citizens of the state well by training people in new fields, conducting research, and communicating closely with its constituents. It is an interdisciplinary program with modern laboratories and expert faculty/scientists. Each faculty member is also a member of a traditional department. The center has close relationships with the colleges of medicine, agriculture, and biological sciences, thus creating strong links that relate researchers to biotechnology. Small groups work on similar projects (e.g., in the neurosciences or plant biotechnology). Such a center fulfills the mission to educate students, conduct research, and interact with the industrial and agricultural organizations in the state. It also generates public support for good public policies. Grass roots support for basic research, incentives for competitive economic projects, improvements in technology infrastructure, modern manufacturing processes, and generation of venture capital can help a great deal in keeping the United States the leader in biotechnology and biomedical research.

References

1. Institute of Medicine. *Careers in Clinical Research—Obstacles and Opportunities*. Washington, DC: National Academy Press; In press.
2. Institute of Medicine. *Careers in Clinical Research*.

CHAPTER V

Innovative Alliances and Commercial Ventures

ABSTRACTS AND EXCERPTS

■ **Adler RG. Genome research: fulfilling the public's expectations for knowledge and commercialization. *Science.* 1992;257:908-914.**

This article provides a historical perspective for the patenting of gene sequences and describes the fundamentals and evolution of patent law. It summarizes federal technology transfer law and policy and assesses the impacts of patenting on academic research. The patentability of gene sequences is then considered along with potential impacts that published sequence data may have on obtaining patent protection for downstream products. Industry's position on gene patenting is summarized and perspectives from the emerging public record on these issues are presented. The article discussing [sic] points at which the filing of patent applications and the licensing of patents may be appropriate. It concludes that technology transfer policies for genome research must be adopted carefully so that they remain viable in a time of rapid technological change.

■ Armstrong JA. University research: new goals, new practices. *Issues in Science and Technology*. 1992-93;IX:50-53.

The end of the Cold War and the increased international competition among national economies is forcing a shift in U.S. priorities, and with it a reevaluation of the rationale for federal support of university research. . . . Many have suggested, . . . that government should refocus its support for research on means of strengthening the nation's welfare and economic competitiveness.

Although it is an issue, and deserves attention, poor technology transfer from the university or national labs to industry has not been a major cause of our competitiveness problem.

There is some danger, therefore, that society at large as well as faculty and administrators will *overstate* what universities can contribute (because they are trying to maximize support) and will consequently do foolish things to the university. . . . people articulate the rationale that we support research because it contributes to commercial competitiveness, there will be tremendous pressure for universities to behave as if they can and should be contributing to competitiveness *in the short term.*

. . . there are a number of ways in which we can improve the rate of return on society's investment in university research without fundamentally harming the ability of universities to create new knowledge and explore new pathways.

Among the areas . . . I will discuss four:

- Improvements in the training of scientists and engineers to enable them to be more effective and enthusiastic participants in the process of R&D exploitation, with a heightened interest in and respect for the intellectual challenges of manufacturing.
- Innovation in the modes of interaction between universities and industry.
- A rationalization of the policies of universities with respect to intellectual property.
- A reexamination, in some cases, of university conflict-of-interest policies and guidelines.

■ Blumenthal D. Academic-industry relationships in the life sciences. *JAMA*. 1992;268:3344-3349.

Academic-industry relationships in the life sciences remain controversial. The available evidence suggests that such relationships have both benefits and risks for involved parties. Benefits include additional support of academic research, income for academic health centers, the potential for increased scientific and commercial productivity in both industries and universities, and enhancement of the educational experiences of students and fellows. Risks include an increase in secrecy in academic environments and damage to public support for the life science enterprise. The balance of known benefits and risks suggests that academic-industry relationships should be permitted and even selectively pro- moted. However, there is also a need for enhanced vigilance on the part of academic institutions and government to reduce risks posed by certain types of arrangements, especially those involving human subjects. Enhanced vigilance should include disclosure of all academic-industry relationships [AIRs] by life science faculty.

The following types of AIRs are among the most common and important, but by no means exhaust the alternatives.

1. Academic-industry research relationships (AIRRs): the support by industry (through grant or contract) of university-based research.
2. Consulting relationships: . . .
3. The sale or licensing of patents by universities to industries: . . .
4. The participation by academic institutions or their faculty in the founding and/or ownership of new companies commercializing university-based research: . . .
5. Academic-industry training relationships: . . .

These and other types of AIRs many occur singly and in combination. The mixed forms of AIRs (such as those involving AIRRs and consulting or equity holding) often raise the most troubling questions of conflict of interest.

■ **Committee on Government Operations.** *Is Science for Sale? Trans-ferring Technology from Universities to Foreign Corporations.* **Washington, D.C.: U.S. Government Printing Office, 1992.**

During the 1980's, there was a dramatic shift among academic scientists to work more closely with industry, partly as a result of Federal legislation designed to speed the transfer of ideas from academia to the marketplace. Closer ties between university researchers and the private sector were encouraged; the goal was to speed the commercialization of new technologies to ensure that the rich intellectual resources developed within our universities would contribute to U.S. economic competitiveness. However, those closer ties have also brought conflicts of interest, where faculty and universities may have a financial interest in the outcome of federally funded research or in the application of the research results by industry. Policy makers therefore need to determine the extent to which research that has been paid for with taxpayers' money should benefit the public, when the public interest conflicts with the university's financial interests or the individual researcher's financial interests.

Conclusions and Recommendations

A. Congress should ensure that research funded by U.S. taxpayers will benefit those taxpayers whenever possible

While technology transfer in and of itself may benefit society, American taxpayers will generally benefit more when American companies are involved, rather than foreign ones.

B. HHS and NSF should give preference to grant applicants who are likely to encourage the application of their research results, and Congress should ensure that American companies have preferential treatment in access to federally funded research results

Despite the frequent rhetoric about the importance of technology transfer, there are few grant programs within HHS or NSF that explicitly specify that preference will be given to applicants who have plans for how to find practical applications for their research results. Such a preference would not always be desirable, but when it is, such preference should be explicitly part of the peer review process.

C. Universities should be required, by statute or regulation, to disclose all links to private companies in grant proposals and disclose in reports whether any foreign companies use their research results

If the agencies do not develop satisfactory regulations in the near future, Congress should require such regulations by statute.

D. Institutions receiving HHS and NSF funds should be required to disclose investments in companies that may benefit from those funds, particularly foreign companies

---

■ Cuatrecasas P. Industry–university alliances in biomedical research. *J Clin Pharmacol.* 1992;32:100-106.

Reprinted with permission of J. B. Lippincott Co.

A recent National Academy of Sciences report proclaimed a "virtual explosion over the past several years in the number and variety of university–industry alliances."

. . . concerns that excessive and inappropriately expressed commercial interests could over time cause adverse and subtle changes on our scholarly institutions are legitimate.

Such concerns must be taken particularly seriously because we are on an irreversible course of changing interrelationships between our business and academic institutions.

. . . it is imperative that as many as possible in the business, university, government and media communities understand the issues and processes involved, and that we all make objective judgements and dispassionate decisions.

. . . a variety of new forces have come together in complex ways to create a fertile ground for new collaborations. Among them are: awareness of foreign competition, encouragement by federal and state agencies, new perceptions of synergies, changes in the state-of-art of the biological sciences, spillover effect of explosion in gene cloning and biotechnology, broader perception of public responsibility of teaching institutions, and demands from customers for more practical results from the research tax dollar.

The fact that the basic or ultimate missions of universities and industry are different does not mean that interactions are incompatible. To the contrary, it can be argued that these are even stronger grounds for collaborating, for sharing and complementing strengths, and for working together to achieve common goals.

In forging a partnership with academia, three areas are particularly troublesome: the concept of applied vs. basic science, the problem of encouraging creativity, and the question of confidentially vs. openness. In these areas, however, the obstacles posed by many critics are largely illusory, and are based on stereotypes, inaccurate definitions, and inexperience.

Industrial laboratories doing fundamental research in the biomedical sciences, with the hope of making discoveries and scientific contributions and uncovering useful new therapeutic agents, are doing work that is intrinsically not so different from that in many university laboratories. They are dealing with the same scientific principles, the same areas of ignorance, the same body of knowledge and theory, and the same challenges of the unknown—so their work cannot be that different, in substance or form. They, too, must hire the best possible scientists, provide them with the environment and resources they need, and assure them of intangible rewards, intellectual outlets, and links of communication to the scientific world. Differences in the nature of the research process are therefore more the function of the behavior of the social institutions within which the work is done.

■ **Eisenberg RS. Genes, patents, and product development.** *Science.* **1992;257:903-908.**

In the past year, the National Institutes of Health (NIH) has filed patent applications on more than 2750 partial complementary DNA sequences of unknown function. The rationale for the filings—that patent protection may be necessary to ensure that private firms are willing to invest in developing related products—rests on two premises: first, that NIH may obtain patent rights that will offer effective product monopolies to licensee firms, and second, that unless NIH obtains these rights now, firms will be unable to obtain a comparable degree of exclusivity by other means, such as by obtaining patents on their own subsequent innovations. Neither premise is clearly wrong, although both are subject to doubt in view of statements from industry representatives that the NIH patenting strategy will deter rather than promote product development.

The Industrial Biotechnology Association (IBA), a trade association whose members collectively represent 80% of U.S. investment in biotechnology, has recently released a position paper urging that NIH not seek patent protection on DNA sequences whose biological function is unknown but instead place such sequences in the public domain.

The paper also expresses concern that patents on partial gene sequences of unknown utility will add to the cost of product development, create a risk of infringement litigation, and encourage companies "to abandon current research efforts that are aimed at product development in favor of routine genetic sequencing for the purpose of staking claims to as much of the genome as possible." The Pharmaceutical Manufacturers Association has taken a similar position in a recent letter to the Secretary of Health and Human Services, expressing the view of its members that "a governmental policy of ownership and licensing of gene sequences would inevitably impede the research and development of new medicines in this country."

Perhaps the bleakest possibility of all from the standpoint of industry is that no one will be able to obtain effective patent protection for genome-related products. It may well be that NIH's disclosure is inadequate to satisfy the enablement standard for the broad claims in the application, yet revealing enough to render subsequent related inventions obvious and therefore unpatentable.

■ Fishbein EA. Ownership of research data. *Academic Medicine.* 1991;66:129-133.

Reprinted with permission of *Academic Medicine* (formerly the *Journal of Medical Education*).

The author reviews the conventional "works for hire" principle that an institution, not its employees, owns the rights to its employees' written products or other forms of expression, including primary research data. This principle is not open to debate as a legal matter. The tough problems giving rise to debates regarding data ownership and access are ethical problems rather than legal ones; these will remain unsettled for some time because at present there is no consensus concerning what constitutes ethical conduct among scholars and scientists and how seriously and in what manner to penalize breaches of that conduct. Access to data is a thorny issue; case histories illustrate the legal and ethical difficulties involved in questions of who has access to information compiled in the course of academic inquiry, and for what purpose. Much depends on the ethics and established procedures of the employing institution, but current case law suggests that a faculty member or institutional researcher does not have any legal right to review the data developed by a colleague. The author recommends that institutions clearly state their policies regarding ownership of data, and presents guidelines for such a policy.

This policy should state in unambiguous terms that:

1. the university or institutional employer asserts its rights to ownership of original primary research data developed by its faculty and employees, regardless of the technology used to create, preserve, or record it;

2. it is the responsibility of faculty members to preserve such data for a stated minimum period of time;

3. the decision to destroy such data must be reviewed and approved by another institutional authority, ...

4. A permanent record must be kept in a centralized place reflecting the inventory of destroyed data, ...

Further, the policy should provide that when investigators depart for other institutions, they normally should be permitted to take copies of research data and related documentary material.

■ Healy B. Special report on gene patenting. *New Engl J Med.* 1992;327:664-668.

Abstracted from information appearing in *NEJM*. Reprinted with permission of the *New England Journal of Medicine*.

A central goal of the Human Genome Project of the National Institutes of Health (NIH) is to accelerate gene discovery by systematically sequencing all 24 unique human chromosomes. There are from 50,000 to 100,000 human genes, and approximately 5000 of them are known to be associated with heritable human traits. Sequencing the genes will create a framework for molecular medical research directed toward an understanding of the genetic bases of human health and disease and of basic life functions, including development.

Recently, Dr. Craig Venter and colleagues at the NIH developed a technique for the rapid sequencing of genes using cDNA, which has made it possible to detect in a few months thousands of previously unknown genes and to obtain partial sequences. Although the approach to gene identification using cDNA is not new, newly developed instrumentation, powerful computers, and advanced robotics have enabled NIH scientists to sequence large segments of expressed genes rapidly.

There are many questions with regard to whether cDNAs should be patentable, and if so, whether the patents should be held by the NIH. Most of these arguments also hold for genomic sequences, which NIH-supported scientists will soon be generating in large numbers.

Should an institution or an individual scientist claim rights to the discovery of a novel molecule when its biologic function is poorly defined? There is a concern that to file for patents for large numbers of partial or full gene sequences with unknown in vivo biologic functions is to seek scientific credit for incomplete discoveries.

Should we patent our "universal heritage"? Some believe that as a matter of social policy, genes—particularly human genes—should not be patented.

Will the patent claims made for cDNA sequences be unfairly broad and too numerous? Some argue that filing a patent application for a fully or partially sequenced gene without having the complete biologic information would be tantamount to claiming the rights to all products resulting from the use of the gene, including the products of gene expression, the antibodies to such products, and any potential uses for them.

Is patenting likely to help or hinder product development?

Should the NIH exert its authority over grantee institutions with respect to cDNA patent filings?

How can international agreement on patent policy best be achieved?

What would happen if all gene-sequence information was placed in the public domain without any protection of intellectual property?

In the face of these many uncertainties, the NIH and the Department of Health and Human Services (DHHS) have adopted a pragmatic interim policy that protects our options and the interests of the taxpayers. This policy preserves options and gives us time to explore thoroughly a series of complex legal, economic, and scientific issues. In brief, we decided to file in order to hold our place. We filed so that we could publish immediately. We filed because no one knows to what degree function must be tied to structure for the patent requirements to be satisfied. In short, we filed to resolve the matter. And while these issues are being resolved through the patent office and through policy discussions nationally and internationally, the patent filing protects U.S. interests.

Despite the criticisms, through the patent application by the NIH we will inevitably move closer to an understanding of how best to translate these rapidly growing numbers of gene-related discoveries into benefits for the public. No outcome is forced by the interim decision of the NIH and the DHHS to file for the patents, and the patent office is in a position to consider an issue of broad relevance.

■ **Kiley TD. Patents on random complementary DNA fragments?** *Science.* **1992;257:915-918.**

The proposal by the National Institutes of Health (NIH) to patent products resulting merely from sequencing the human genome is a mistake: at worst, it is wrong in patent law; at best, it relies on deficiencies in law concerning what is "useful" as a requirement for patents. The proposal is symptomatic of a problem besieging biotechnology—attempts to control the raw material of scientific experimentation before research has determined the practical value of such material—that needs curing on many fronts. Corrective measures are proposed for adoption by the Executive branch, the Congress, and the courts.

The Patent and Trademark Office (PTO) should expedite review of the NIH patent applications, reject them for failure to meet the *Brenner v. Manson* standard, and expedite appeal from the rejection to the Court of Appeals for the Federal Circuit, where all interested parties can make their views known by learned briefs amici curiae.

Congress should change law that now permits research efforts that use patented inventions to be shut down. The object would be to free scientific research wherever it gets done from the threat of foreclosure by injunction. The new criterion for injunction should be whether an already patented invention is itself placed into the stream of commerce, as distinct from its being used en route to the invention of a different thing.

To provide NIH the full benefit of the public debate it aims to sponsor, the Executive branch should ensure that the NIH applications and proceedings in the PTO concerning them remain open to public view.

Finally, let the Executive branch now seek to change federal law to ensure that agencies can prohibit patents on inventions made by their employees where, after due process, the agency determines those are not in the public interest.

■ **Mansfield E. Academic research and industrial innovation.** *Research Policy.* **1991;20:1-12. (See also Mansfield E. Academic research and industrial innovation: A further note.** *Research Policy.* **1992;21:295-296.)**

The purpose of this study is to estimate the extent to which technological innovations in various industries have been based on recent academic research, and the time lags between the investment in recent academic research projects and the industrial utilization of their findings. Because no attempt (to my knowledge) has been made to estimate the social rate of return from academic research, we also make some rough and tentative estimates of this sort. While the results are subject to many limitations discussed below, they should be of interest to public policy-makers concerned with science and technology, as well as to economists and others that study the process of technological change.

Because the results of academic research are so widely disseminated and their effects are so fundamental, subtle, and widespread, it is difficult to identify and measure the links between academic research and industrial innovation. This paper presents, apparently for the first time, data concerning the percentage of new products and processes that, according to the innovating firms, could not have been developed (without substantial delay) in the absence of recent academic research.

. . . our results provide convincing evidence that, particularly in industries like drugs, instruments, and information processing, the contribution of academic research to industrial innovation has been considerable. . . . Our results, while they do not address the very difficult question of how to allocate the social returns between academic and industrial research, indicate that, without recent academic research, there would have been a substantial reduction in social benefits.

To prevent misunderstanding, it may be worthwhile to conclude by recognizing that the rationale for academic research extends far beyond the sorts of narrowly defined economic benefits considered here. Obviously, knowledge concerning the universe is important for its own sake, and the education of students, which occurs in many academic research projects, is socially important as well. Nonetheless, it is interesting to find that, even if academic research is judged in these relatively restricted terms, its role seems to be substantial.

■ **Moriarty CM, Purdy JB. University research: planning for the 1990s.** *Educational Record.* **1992;Summer:51-56.**

Reprinted with permission of the authors.

The research community may be surprised to learn that insufficient funding is *not* the biggest problem if faces today. . . . the American research community's most troublesome problem is its lack of clearly defined priorities.

Historically, universities have invested little effort in proactive planning, particularly when it has involved research. . . . But proactive planning has become essential to a prosperous research program. Research university administrators must develop and refine strategies to help their institutions thrive in the coming decade and beyond. . . . They will certainly encounter pressures and prospects that will restrict their efforts, and they will grapple with a host of difficult issues...:

- how (or whether) to maintain a broad research base in a climate of increasing costs and highly specialized equipment that regularly and rapidly becomes obsolete, and accompanied by a diminishing pool of talented faculty;
- whether (or how) to adopt a corporate model and establish a "market niche" to enhance and expand specific elements of institutional uniqueness; and
- how to make changes without corrupting the mission and culture of the university.

. . . the research initiatives proposed as a part of the overall plan should include:

- the endorsement of appropriate department heads and deans, and identification of local support committed to the initiative.
- Identification of how the proposal will benefit the university's research program and its potential for future growth.
- The impact that the proposed initiative will have on existing programs.
- A defensible budget, with projections for the out-years. (Space needs, if any, should be addressed.)
- The potential and plan(s) for acquiring long-term funding if and when institutional funds are either phased out or reduced to baseline levels.

■ Mowery DC. The U.S. national innovation system: origins and prospects for change. *Research Policy*. 1992;21:125-144.

Reprinted with permission of Elsevier Science Publishers B.V.

This paper examines the origins and outlook for the features of the U.S. national innovation system that have historically distinguished this system from those of other industrial economies. Among these features are (1) the prominent role of antitrust policy; (2) the large share of postwar national R&D expenditures accounted for by government and, within the national governmental R&D budget, the large defense share; and (3) during the postwar period, the significant role of relatively small, new firms in the commercialization of new technologies. The new international economic and technological environment has given rise to a domestic debate over U.S. technology policy that in combination with these elements of change may significantly alter these distinguishing features of the U.S. innovation system.

Predictions about "the future of the U.S. innovation system" are hazardous at best, not least because the complex institutional array that affects the innovative performance of the U.S. economy can scarcely be described as a system established with any explicit economic objectives in mind. If nothing else, this paper should show the extent to which several of the unique characteristics of the U.S. innovation system were in fact unintended effects of public policies (e.g., antitrust or military procurement) formulated with little if any consideration of their effects on the innovative performance of the overall economy. Moreover, many current U.S. initiatives or proposals that respond to political demands for a "civilian technology strategy" formulated with such economic objectives in mind seemingly wish to deny the growing interdependence among ostensibly "national" innovation systems. These policies may themselves yield significant unintended consequences. As such, "convergence" in the structure of the innovation systems of the U.S. and other industrial economies is likely to be halting, unplanned, and slow to develop.

■ Rosenberg N. Scientific instrumentation and university research. *Research Policy.* 1992;21:381-390.

The purpose of this paper is to examine certain roles played by the American research university in the development of an important category of technology: scientific instruments.

. . . much of the scientific instrumentation that is now in existence had its historical origins in the conduct of basic research—specifically, in the attempt to advance the frontier of scientific knowledge through an expansion in observational or experimental capabilities. In this sense, a central part of the "output" of the university research enterprise has been much more than just new theories explaining some aspect of the structure of the universe or additional data confirming or modifying existing theories. An additional output (or byproduct) has been more powerful and more versatile techniques of instrumentation including, in many cases, an ability to observe or measure phenomena that were previously not observable or measurable at all. In this sense, new instrumentation has often been an unintentional and, to a surprising extent, even an unacknowledged, product of university research.

Instrumentation and techniques have moved from one scientific discipline to another in ways that have been very consequential for the progress of science. . . . The flow appears to have been particularly heavy from physics to chemistry, as well as from both physics and chemistry to biology, to clinical medicine, and ultimately to health care delivery.

Many instrumentation technologies that originated in university laboratories have eventually been taken up, produced and sold by profit-making firms. This has typically resulted in great improvements in performance and versatility as well as reductions in the price of the product. This aspect of commercialization has meant, in turn, that the instrument has become much more widely diffused throughout both industry and the university research community that originally gave rise to it. This process has vastly expanded the size of the industrial and research populations to which the instrumentation was accessible. . . . Thus, the ultimate benefits have flowed not only to the industrial world, but in some considerable measure back to a much larger scientific research community whose members have been provided with greater access to improved instrumentation.

. . . the need for improved instrumentation has had consequences far beyond those that are indicated by thinking of them simply as an expanding class of devices that are useful for observation and measurement. I am also suggesting that they have played much more pervasive, if less visible roles, which included a direct effect upon industrial capabilities, on the one hand, and the stimulation of more scientific research, on the other. This even includes a role of great importance in redefining and expanding the agenda of fundamental university research.

It is possible to go a step farther. It follows from what has been said that the rate of progress, and the timing of progress, in individual scientific disciplines may be shaped, to a considerable degree, by the transfer of instruments, experimental techniques and concepts from one scientific discipline to another.

■ **United States General Accounting Office.** *University Research: Controlling Inappropriate Access to Federally Funded Research Results.* **Washington, D.C.: United States General Accounting Office, 1992.**

The importance of university research to technological innovation increased dramatically during the 1980s, creating new linkages among the academic community, industry, and the federal government. . . . However, closer ties between universities and businesses raise concern about possible conflicts of interest or other relationships that might give a business inappropriate access to, and therefore an unfair advantage in commercializing, the results of federally funded research.

. . . we examine these linkages by surveying the principal universities receiving funding from the National Institutes of Health (NIH) and the National Science Foundation (NSF).

During fiscal years 1989 and 1990, the 35 universities we surveyed granted 536 licenses and received $82 million in income for technologies developed in whole or in part with NIH or NSF funding.

Twenty-four universities had industrial liaison programs with at least one foreign company member. Fourteen of these universities reported that industrial liaison program members can get advance access to the results of federally funded research before the results are made generally available. NIH and NSF guidelines do not address the extent to which program members can be given such advance access.

Relationships between licensees and universities are becoming increasingly complex. The 35 universities reported that (1) scientists who developed the technologies for 61 exclusive licenses consulted for, owned a substantial amount of stock in, or had other relationships with the licensees and (2) members of industrial liaison programs were granted exclusive licenses in four cases.

Conclusions

Requiring that investigators and other key personnel disclose certain types of outside interests as part of the grant award process, which both NIH and NSF are considering, is an essential first step for improving university management controls over potential conflicts of interest.

We recommend that the Secretary of Health and Human Services and the Director of NSF require that their grantees have procedures in place to effectively manage potential conflicts of interest. . . . We also recommend that NIH and NSF review their funding recipients' policies and procedures to ensure that they adequately address conflicts-of-interest issues. Furthermore, we recommend that NIH and NSF develop policies that address the extent to which U.S. and foreign industrial liaison program members can be given advance access to research the agencies have funded.

COMMENTARY

Leslie Cutler

Should academic institutions form alliances with business and industry to enhance innovation and commercialization? Are such alliances needed and, if so, why are they necessary? Is it time to change the traditional separation between the conduct of "basic research," which has been primarily the province of universities, and "applied research and development," which has been the domain of business and industry? These are questions that are being asked with increasing frequency as America struggles to compete economically in the global marketplace.

Concurrently, there is an increasing call by economists, business and government leaders, and the public to make federally funded research more relevant to society's goals. This is articulated in Rep. George E. Brown, Jr.'s 1992 *Chairman's Report of the Task Force on the Health of Research* to the House Committee on Science, Space, and Technology, where he enunciated the position that the nation's investment in science, especially university-based, fundamental research, is not leading to the economic and societal benefits the country needs to maintain and improve our quality of life and to remain competitive in the international marketplace.

While these assumptions may, to some extent, be correct, the core of the problem is not with our system of basic research. Over the past several years numerous articles have pointed out that our international competitors have captured various consumer product markets through the process of incremental improvements on the design and manufacturing of inventions made in America. These articles have pointed to both the short-term financial objectives which many U.S. firms and industries use to guide their approach to management and the relative lack of investment in research and development to improve either products or manufacturing processes. Indeed, U.S. industry only directs about 20 percent of its

R&D investments towards long-term goals. In contrast, our Japanese and European competitors invest 50 to 60 percent of their research funds in long-term R&D.

By way of contrast, the U.S. pharmaceutical and the related biotechnology industries have maintained their long-term approach to R&D and close ties with university-based research. It is no surprise that we are the world leaders in these industries. However, our foreign competitors are aggressively seeking to capture these industries while our own government is reducing funding for basic science and initiating regulations to constrain the commercial interaction between universities and our partners in these industries.

Many analysts have concluded that, in contrast to their skills at incremental improvement, our foreign competitors are not very accomplished at inventing and developing new ideas. Some would agree that while the Japanese, for example, excel in their ability to improve on existing products and methods, they have not been pioneers. The Japanese must still master the tasks of inventing new products, markets, and even whole businesses.

How will Japan and other international competitors master these more daunting tasks? The answer is simple. These countries are buying, or trying to buy, the best basic research minds and the best research system in the world. They are, in fact, trying to buy the research infrastructure of the United States, the very system that many people in Congress and elsewhere are trying to change.

The Nippon Electronic Corporation's new laboratory in Princeton, New Jersey, employs 40 of our nation's best scientists to study fundamental problems in physics and computer science. Hitachi has built a multimillion-dollar research center on the campus of the University of California, Irvine, and many of the molecular and cell biologists working in the building are employees of the Hitachi Chemical Research Center, Inc. Significant portions of many of the best university spinoff biotechnology companies are now owned by foreign companies; Sandoz, the Swiss pharmaceutical company, recently structured a lucrative and controversial licensing arrangement with the Scripps Institute in La Jolla, California.

It is worth reiterating: The marketplace and our international competitors have identified the U.S. system of university-based, fundamental research, especially those portions related to biotechnology and biomedical research, as the research enterprise that is most likely to yield the knowledge, ideas, and inventions that will lead to marketable products for the future. This is a system which is founded on taking the long-term approach to science. It is a system which incrementally explores and builds on each basic discovery, a system proven to create the information needed to serve as the foundation upon which valuable products and processes can be developed. The success of this system rests on practices and philosophies which are distinctly different from those which drive much of the U.S. business community.

The structure of the current relationships between the university-based research enterprise and industry is not working optimally for business, the university community, or the country. To succeed in the future, we must invent a new paradigm for the interaction between universities and industry. We must create a balanced system in which basic science and the incremental improvements on the discoveries of this science that are necessary to bring high-quality, cost-competitive products to market are conducted conjointly. An active process for structuring alliances between the scholarly community and business is required. This should be one that facilitates the innovation and commercialization of products which help achieve the nation's economic and social agendas without damaging the purpose, principles, and qualities of the academy.

The development of such alliances can add value to both enterprises. Industry can benefit by being closer to the source of the basic science and by adopting some of the long-term perspectives of the academic community. The university research enterprise can benefit not only from seeing the rapid incorporation of basic science into products and services that help the nation socially and financially, but also by learning how to look for more rapid, cost-effective methods to develop basic knowledge. We must realize that the university research community can facilitate the transfer of research findings and take part in commercialization without sacrificing the community's principles or goals.

In summary, the U.S. economy may continue to falter, and the perception of and belief in the value of independent, university-based fundamental science will decline if we do not change the paradigm governing the interaction of the university research community and industry. The initial signs of the need for change are already evident. The data that indicate that we can succeed by taking a new, allied approach are strong. We, in the academy and in industry, must form collegial, organized, cost-effective, efficient alliances. We must capitalize on each other's unique strengths to enhance basic science and the development of innovative products and processes that meet society's needs and are commercially successful in the global marketplace.

COMMENTARY

Cynthia Maurer-Sutton and William N. Kelley

The United States needs to encourage the transfer of technology that is discovered in our research laboratories in order to optimize the benefits of science for the American people. One way to facilitate this technology transfer is through the development of joint relationships between universities and industry. These joint relationships can take on many different forms, including but not limited to industry-sponsored research, consulting agreements between researchers and industry, license agreements between academe and industry, university ownership positions in new start-ups, joint appointments of researchers to both industry and academe, joint recruitment of post-doctoral fellows and graduate students, and industry liaison programs.

There is convincing evidence, particularly in the pharmaceutical and similar industries, that the contribution of academic research to industrial innovation has been considerable. Without recent academic research there would have been a substantial reduction in social benefits. As funding becomes more difficult to obtain from traditional sources, the relationships with industry are going to become more important to the academic health centers to continue their research programs. Cuatrecasas notes that while federal funding levels have been moderating, corporate contributions to academic research have increased more than three-fold between 1980 and 1987, and totaled nearly $700 million in 1987 alone. However, it is important to note that federal funding is still significantly greater for the same time period, approximately $7 billion.

There are a number of ways to improve the rate of return on society's investment to university research without fundamentally harming the ability of universities to create new knowledge and explore new pathways. One way is to provide support for the identification and training of clinical investigators. With the pace at which knowledge in biomedicine is being developed, there is a tremendous need to attract the best candidates to become trained physician-scientists who will transform medical discoveries into effective treatments for human disease. In addition, we need to revise the training of these scientists not only to be more effective and enthusiastic participants in technology transfer but also to respect the intellectual challenges of development and manufacturing. Academe must overcome a bias that favors pure science over applied science.

Second, innovative ways need to be developed to improve the interactions between university faculty and industrial scientists. In developing these modes of interaction, we must ensure that each party has an understanding and agreement on the intellectual property issues in addition to having appropriate conflict-of-interest policies to guide them in their decision making.

There are several forces that make this the right time to develop innovative methods to improve the interaction between academe and industry. First, the ability to identify disease genes by a new technology termed "positional cloning" in combination with the strategic efforts to fully map the human genome is quickly bringing us to a point where it will be possible to define the exact genetic basis for every human disease. This explosion of new information will allow full application of new therapeutic modalities, including chemical, biological, and most recently, genetic therapies. The opportunities for translating information from molecular biology to the health care delivery arena have never been greater.[1] Secondly, biomedical research and the transfer of technology to the marketplace are extremely important to the health and welfare of the American people and our nation's global competitiveness. Finally, the American people, who are the customers for government research, are asking for practical results from the research that is funded by their tax dollars.

Thus the debate is not whether we need university-industry relationships, but how we can enhance these relationships and maximize the results of these ties. The benefits of university-industry relationships include the direct financial support of academic research, the potential for increased scientific and commercial productivity in both industries and universities, and the enhancement of the educational experience of students and fellows. Some people say that we need to regulate these relationships when the public interest conflicts with either the university's or the researcher's financial interests. However, the public's interest is the best way to support an effective and efficient technology transfer process. If universities have appropriate conflict-of-interest policies, the government should not add a layer of bureaucracy that is not needed and may cause a negative impact on the effectiveness and efficiency of the transfer of the technology.

In order to appropriately develop the university-industry relationship in an academic health center, it is important to recognize the potential risks associated with these relationships and develop mechanisms to minimize them. A frequently mentioned concern is the potential for increased secrecy and thus limitations on publishing of important findings resulting from research being performed in academe. This can be addressed through the development of appropriate institutional policies, which are then conveyed through contracts with industry, that limit the amount of time industry has to review a particular finding prior to publishing by the faculty member. A second area often noted is the potential for a lack of emphasis on teaching and neglect of basic research. Both of these issues can be addressed through the appropriate mechanisms for advancement and recognition within the Medical School. Another point often raised is that university-industry relationships might influence the academician to undertake research that would have commercial application. By avoiding excessive dependence on industry research support, especially with one company, and by having in place the correct guidelines for advancement as referenced above, this risk can also be managed. And finally one of the major areas of concern is the potential for conflict-of-interest issues. It is a shame that the relationships that have significant potential conflict-of-interest issues have received a majority of the publicity as compared to the large number of relationships that are appropriately developed and executed. In addition, the number of questionable deals to acceptable deals appears, likewise, to be quite small. Nevertheless, it is important to develop mechanisms within academia and industry to address these issues and minimize their occurrence.

University-industry relationships have documented benefits which provide a persuasive argument for continuing and, in fact, enhancing these relationships. In order to address the concerns raised and enhance these joint relationships, public policy should consider the following recommendations:

(1) Universities should avoid an excessive dependance on industrial relationships for research support, especially with one company providing a majority of the research support. Using the financial investment model as an example to follow, universities should diversify their portfolios of research funding to many different organizations, including the government and industry, to maximize their return on investment.

(2) It is neither practical nor desirable for the federal government to dictate detailed rules for the management of university-industry relationships. However, it is appropriate for the government to require all institutional grantees to develop a process through which university-industry relationships of federally supported researchers are disclosed and reviewed in

a confidential manner by academic officials. In addition, the federal government should neither fund clinical research if the principal investigator has a personal financial relationship with the company that may be affected by the outcome of research nor any research where the personal financial interest in the company affects the outcome of the research.

(3) Academic institutions should require regular (i.e., at least annual) disclosure by faculty of their outside interests, or significant financial relationships to any companies. In addition, prior to any negotiations for a university-industry arrangement, the involved faculty member should disclose any of his or her financial ties to the company. If the faculty member does have a financial relationship with a company it should be governed by the institution's conflict-of-interest policy referenced below.

(4) Academic institutions should develop guidelines for developing appropriate university-industry relationships, and these guidelines should be evaluated on a periodic basis to ensure appropriateness, compliance, and future applicability.

(5) Academic institutions need to develop conflict-of-interest policies that address among other things, a faculty member's participation with industry. These policies should include a mechanism to address potential conflict-of-interest issues because there will always be some potential conflict-of-interest issues, whether actual or perceived. The solution becomes how best to manage the issues to minimize the risks. We have found that there needs to be a conflict-of-interest committee that meets in a timely fashion to address issues that are specific to each case that comes before the committee. After an analysis of each case, the committee provides recommendations to the faculty member and administration on how to minimize the perceived risks of conflict of interest.

(6) The administration of academic institutions should be negotiating the arrangements with industry. Each alliance should be developed to minimize the potential risks discussed above. Special attention should be given to analysis of the arrange-

ment when more than one relationship with a company (e.g., research and license agreements) occurs.

Reference

1. Institute of Medicine Report. *Careers in Clinical Research—Obstacles and Opportunities.* Washington, DC: National Academy Press; in press.

CHAPTER VI

Integrity in Scientific Research

ABSTRACTS AND EXCERPTS

■ Institute of Medicine. *Responsible Science: Ensuring the Integrity of the Research Process*, Volume I. Washington, D.C.: National Academy Press, 1992:1-16.

Comparatively recent and dramatic increases in the size and influence of the U.S. research enterprise, and in the amounts and patterns of funding, have led to changing social expectations about the accountability of scientists and their institutions for research supported by public funds. In addition, the changing nature of collaborative efforts, the quickening pace and increasing complexity of research endeavors, and the growing emphasis on commercialization of research results have combined to exacerbate stresses that have always been apparent to some extent in scientific research. During the last decade, reports of wrongdoing in science have been accompanied by government oversight and continued scrutiny of the conduct of scientific research. All of these developments have profound implications for the research enterprise's system of internal checks and balances, which evolved in a research environment far removed from the forces of the political process.

To address concerns that affect the entire U.S. scientific community, the Committee on Science, Engineering, and Public Policy (COSEPUP) of the National Academy of Sciences, the National Academy of Engineering, and the Institute of

Medicine convened the 22-member Panel on Scientific Responsibility and the Conduct of Research. The panel was asked to examine the following issues:

1. What is the state of current knowledge about modern research practices for a range of disciplines, including trends and practices that could affect the integrity of research?

2. What are the advantages and disadvantages of enhanced educational efforts and explicit guidelines for researchers and research institutions? Can the research community itself define and strengthen basic standards for scientists and their institutions?

3. What roles are appropriate for public and private institutions in promoting responsible research practices? What can be learned from institutional experiences with current procedures for handling allegations of misconduct in science?

. . . the panel was also asked to determine whether existing unwritten practices should be expressed as principles to guide the responsible conduct of research. If the panel members judged it advisable, they were encouraged to prepare model guidelines and other materials.

Ensuring the integrity of the research process requires that scientists and research institutions give systematic attention to the fundamental values, principles, and traditions that foster responsible research conduct. In considering factors that may affect integrity and misconduct in science, the panel formulated twelve recommendations to strengthen the research enterprise and to clarify the nature of the responsibilities of scientists, research institutions, and government agencies in this area.

Recommendation One

Individual scientists in cooperation with officials of research institutions should accept formal responsibility for ensuring the integrity of the research process.

Recommendation Two

Scientists and research institutions should integrate into their curricula educational programs that foster faculty and student awareness of concerns related to the integrity of the research process.

Recommendation Three

Adoption of formal guidelines for the conduct of research. . . should be an option, not a requirement, for research institutions.

Recommendation Four

Research institutions and government agencies should adopt a common framework of definitions, distinguishing among misconduct in science, questionable research practices, and other forms of misconduct.

Recommendation Five

Government agencies should adopt common policies and procedures for handling allegations of misconduct in science.

Recommendation Six

Research institutions and government research agencies should have policies and procedures that ensure appropriate and prompt responses to allegations of misconduct in science.

Recommendation Seven

Scientists and their institutions should act to discourage questionable research practices through a broad range of formal and informal methods in the research environment.

Recommendation Eight

Research institutions should have policies and procedures to address other misconduct—such as theft, harassment, or vandalism—that may occur in the research environment.

Recommendation Nine

Government research agencies should clarify their roles in addressing misconduct in science, questionable research practices, and other misconduct.

Recommendation Ten

An independent Scientific Integrity Advisory Board should be created by the scientific community and research institutions to exercise leadership in addressing ethical issues in research conduct;

Recommendation Eleven

The important role that individual scientists can play in disclosing incidents of misconduct in science should be acknowledged.

Recommendation Twelve

Scientific societies and scientific journals should continue to provide and expand resources and forums to foster responsible research practices and to address misconduct in science and questionable research practices.

■ **Maechling C. The laboratory is not a courtroom.** *Issues in Science & Technology.* **1992;8:73-77.**

. . . despite scientists' contention that cases of blatant plagiarism and falsification of research data or results are comparatively rare, allegations of misconduct continue to surface. In response, the National Institutes of Health and the National Science Foundation have each promulgated new procedures for investigating and punishing misconduct in federally funded research projects. These regulations place the primary responsibility for dealing with misconduct allegations on the research institutions concerned; only if the latter fail to take prompt and effective action, or if criminal charges emerge, will government investigative bodies take over.

Eager to protect the autonomy of the scientific enterprise and avert government intervention, universities and other recipients of federal research funds have moved quickly to adopt more structured investigative and disciplinary procedures than were formerly customary in an academic environment. Unfortunately, by using U.S. trial procedure as a model, these research institutions have unwittingly allowed many of the undesirable features of the adversarial system on which this procedure is based to be smuggled in under the benign mantle of "due process." This is distorting the delicate task of investigating questionable research practices and could do lasting damage to the health of U.S. science.

The inquisitorial or civil law system, which is derived from Roman law, offers an alternative model that provides a much closer fit to traditional academic procedures.

The main feature of civil-law trial procedure that makes it so appropriate for a misconduct inquiry is that it does not in principle start out with an "accused." The initial focus is on the alleged crime and its circumstances. Only if a suspect emerges from an assessment of the evidence will the investigation center on the person responsible.

. . . the spirit of objective inquiry during the investigative or examination phase provides greater protection for the individual than the adversarial model with its prosecutorial approach and spotlight on accuser and accused.

. . . the prospects for eradicating misconduct will not be improved by inflaming the scientific environment and clogging investigative challenges with adversarial procedures imported from the criminal justice system. The cultures of law and scientific research are radically different—one is devoted to selective exploitation of facts for specific ends, the other to exploration of the unknown; they should not be confused. Universities and private research institutions should stick with their traditional method of objective inquiry by qualified scientific peers.

■ **Pellegrino ED. Character and the ethical conduct of research.** *Accountability in Research.* **1992;2:1-11.**

Recurrent disclosure of scientific fraud, conflict of interest and other forms of misconduct have cast a shadow over the moral integrity of the research enterprise. Congress and the public are asking seriously if science can be left to govern itself. There are forebodings in current Congressional investigations of serious legal and regulatory constraints on the conduct of research. The integrity of science and the benefits of research to society are seriously threatened.

If research is to be safeguarded against these eventualities the onus of responsibility rests with the scientific community. It must give evidence of its moral probity. Rather than denying or trivializing misconduct, we must accept moral accountability for it. Rather than demanding freedom we must earn it. We must confront the ineluctable fact that the scientific community holds its freedom and support in trust. If that freedom is abused all science and scientists are morally diminished and society may justly intervene.

Even in today's complicated milieu of industrialization, commercialization and corporatization of research the final determinant of the quality of research remains character and conscience of the scientists. We must return to the ethics of personal responsibility, the most ancient branch of ethics, the ethics of character and virtue. Paradoxically by taking the moral high road even at the risk of non-survival, we take the surest way to survival.

■ Shimm DS, Spece RG. Industry reimbursement for entering patients into clinical trials: legal and ethical issues. *Annals of Internal Medicine.* 1991;115:148-151.

Reprinted with permission of the *Annals of Internal Medicine*.

Pharmaceutical manufacturers commonly contract with clinical investigators for pre-market testing of new products. The per-patient reimbursement offered to the investigator generally exceeds the per-patient costs incurred by the investigator. This excess represents a windfall that can be used to pay for travel, equipment, or supplies, or to fund research for which the investigator cannot obtain funding through peer-reviewed granting channels. This excess raises a potential conflict of interest, because it may lead the investigator to propose experimental treatment for a patient when the patient might be better served by conventional treatment or by no treatment at all. Not only does this situation pose a conflict of interest, it also is a conflict of which few patients are aware and fewer are informed. We propose that all experimental subjects be informed of the source, amount, and mechanism of funding for the experimental treatments they undergo.

Further, we propose that payments from pharmaceutical manufacturers for pre-market testing of drugs go to the medical school dean rather than to the individual investigator. With this money, the dean can defray the direct as well as the indirect costs of the clinical study; the remainder, which would otherwise go directly to the investigator, should be placed in a funding pool for which the entire medical school could compete.

This solution largely eliminates conflict of interest, addresses informed consent, and reasonably balances the interests of the experimental subject, the clinical investigator, the pharmaceutical manufacturer, and the academic institution.

COMMENTARY

John F. Griffith with F. Daniel Davis

My friend and colleague, Edmund Pellegrino, argues in his essay, "Character and the Ethical Conduct of Research," that the character and virtue of the individual scientist provide the most secure anchors to protect integrity and guard against misconduct in research. In the brief remarks that follow, I wish to underscore the critical role of the mentoring relationship in the formation of scientific integrity, which is essential to the pursuit of truth, the central objective of science. The senior scientist is obligated to provide the exemplar of professional integrity—to teach and cultivate integrity by example—to the young investigator who is just beginning to acquire the methods, skills, and values demanded by this pursuit. The late Nobel laureate John F. Enders carried out this obligation with the utmost care, diligence, and devotion. My strong convictions about mentoring reflect, in part, my own experience of working under his tutelage.

I will argue, then, that in the mentoring relationship with the senior scientist, the character of the young scientist qua scientist is developed and formed. Rules, principles, and procedures may help to guide the pursuit of scientific knowledge and truth, but it is in and through the mentoring relationship that young scientists acquire the most effective, often the most lasting moral compass, by observing and internalizing the examples of their mentors. The importance of the mentoring relationship for integrity in research has been obscured, however, and its role has been diminished by several tendencies evident in science today. These tendencies present a real challenge to scientists, senior and junior alike, and represent less than optimal conditions for instilling and cultivating the values essential to science. To master these challenges, we must first recognize them as such, and then find concrete ways to reaffirm and strengthen the role of the mentoring relationship in ensuring the integrity of the individual scientist and the scientific enterprise as a whole.

In recent years we have witnessed an increasingly intense focus on both alleged and proven scientific misconduct. The uproar over allegations against some of the luminaries of contemporary science, the glare of the media spotlight, and the acrimonious hearings before congressional committees all imply within and beyond the scientific community that something is amiss with science today. Has scientific misconduct become the kind of pervasive phenomenon suggested in the newspapers and in the halls of Congress? Is scientific integrity currently in eclipse?

We have no way of reliably determining the incidence of scientific misconduct, either now or then, regardless of how one defined "then." Above all else, science is a human endeavor. As such, it always has been—and always will be—marred from time to time by the all-too-human frailties of dishonesty, laxity, and selfishness. Compared to the sheer number of investigations funded by public and private agencies, however, the number of reported allegations of scientific misconduct is actually very small. Nonetheless, it is important to explore any possible connection between the emergence of scientific misconduct as a controversial problem on the one hand and the state of contemporary science on the other.

One of the more striking differences between the science a few decades ago and science today is the difference between small and large. Today, research is often conducted in a large laboratory, which is usually dominated by a senior scientist or principal investigator, and populated by many pre- and post-doctoral trainees and technicians. The setting is also highly bureaucratized due to complex fiscal, technological, and administrative arrangements. Managing these arrangements, writing new grant applications, and overseeing experiments and the production of papers are activities that demand much of the senior investigator's time and energy. Indeed, for life in the large laboratory, which seems to be emerging as the paradigmatic setting for research, a management or business degree is just as relevant as a doctoral degree in one of the sciences.

The definition of scientists as scholars and mentors, first and foremost, has been somewhat blurred by the imperative to manage the laboratory as though it were a factory. In light of the intense pressures to "publish or perish," the material rewards that scientific achievement can bring, and the heated competition for scientific funding, there should be little surprise that the scientific laboratory of today is often just that, a factory. In this setting, junior scientists often find themselves somewhat adrift, with only brief contact rather than ongoing, meaningful dialogue with their mentors. Instruction in highly technical methods and procedures for investigation is often a responsibility dispersed among older students and technicians. Time is often in short supply for a substantive mentoring relationship and for the critical give-and-take through which science—and its values—are taught and learned.

In the practice of contemporary science, there are, of course, exceptions to these tendencies; there are still examples of the kind of mentoring relationship that I enjoyed with Enders several decades ago. "The Chief," as he was affectionately known in the laboratory, was the embodiment of scientific integrity; many of his personal characteristics and habits seem, at least to me, to exemplify this quality. He spent most of his time in the laboratory and very little attending out-of-town meetings. Thus, more often than not, he was available to his students and trainees to discuss and challenge our ideas about research directions as well as the accuracy and reproducibility of our findings. He brought his considerable intelligence, skill, and experience to bear on every dimension of an investigation, from beginning to end. The way one designed an experiment, recorded or interpreted data, and worded a grant proposal or manuscript was carefully, but unflinchingly, critiqued by the Chief, who demanded that everyone in his laboratory become "one's own best critic."

Enders did not attach his name to every publication that originated from his laboratory, even though he contributed to every experiment; he included himself as an author only when his contribution was major. Quite simply, he was an extremely honest person with exceptionally high standards. At the same time, he was uniquely modest, particularly in light of the scientific and public acclaim he received for his epic work with the polio and measles viruses. His performance standards surpassed the threshold of external peer review, because he insisted on knowing the details and being aware of all work in progress. In summary, scientific integrity was a constant agenda in Enders' laboratory, not because of the Office of Scientific Integrity of the National Institutes of Health or the scrutiny of the Congress, but because the Chief explicitly assumed responsibility for such integrity. In the final analysis, unless those who are responsible for research laboratories and the training of future investigators behave more like Enders, scientific integrity or the lack thereof, will remain a problem.

Neither my arguments nor my reflections have yielded a definitive description of the link between the contemporary state of science and the problems of scientific integrity or misconduct. I am arguing, however, that many of the tendencies that now prevail in science—and, for that matter, in medicine—represent a real challenge to the mentoring relationship and thus to the *ethical* practice of these professions. This allusion to parallels between the ethics of science and the ethics of medicine naturally arises within the setting of an academic health center, where medicine and science are pursued not only in close proximity to one another but also in overlapping ways. Medicine, like science, is increasingly depersonalized and bureaucratized. That fact, however, only makes it all the more necessary that we be aware of the importance of the mentoring relationship in both medicine and science. For just as young investigators look to senior scientists as models of integrity in research, medical students and residents look to attending physicians as exemplars of "good" medicine. And "good" in this sense means scientifically *and* ethically "good." Without sound models and without proper mentoring, young investigators and physicians can become susceptible to the pressures and tendencies that now beset these professions.

Since the days of Hippocrates, physicians—and one could add here, scientists as well—have been guided by a spirit of generosity toward their students. The most secure anchor for integrity in science and medicine is the character and virtue of an individual such as John Enders, whose life and work exemplified the ideals of generosity, honesty, and critical intelligence. In addition to affirming the importance of the mentoring relationship as the context in which integrity takes root and develops, academic institutions should redouble their efforts to emphasize quality, not quantity, in scientific research.

Deans and other administrators should sharpen their focus on what constitutes productivity and accomplishment. For example, they should read papers rather than simply weighing curricula vitaes. Quality work may mean a single study that is thoroughly done and results in an important publication which shapes the thinking of others. If in the service of quantity rather than quality, young investigators acquire bad habits, cut corners, and publish superficially then scientific integrity and misconduct will, indeed, be problematic. The solutions are simple but fairly complex.

COMMENTARY

Michael E. Johns and David A. Blake

Particularly evident in biomedical research is the concomitance of opportunities and threats. This promising but relatively young field of science has seen its integrity questioned repeatedly and publicly over the past decade. Widely heralded cases of scientific fraud and other forms of scientific misconduct have been regular features in the national press. The appearance of conflicts of interest has resulted from linkages that faculty and academic institutions have to the commercial sector. Furthermore, the ability of universities to keep their academic houses in order has been called into question.

Major discoveries of the molecular genetics basis for diseases with the attendant potential for curative genetic therapies are becoming weekly events. Through incredible new imaging technologies, neuroscientists literally have a window on the brain and its functions. These dazzling discoveries are attracting the interest of the brightest youth and the support of a wide range of research sponsors. Threats to the integrity of biomedical research are particularly unfortunate during an unprecedented era of opportunities in molecular medicine and neurosciences. Therefore, if this great promise is to be realized, integrity in the biomedical research enterprise must be restored and maintained. The primary responsibility rests with the academic institutions that train the next generation of scientists. However, it is one thing for institutions to claim primary responsibility for maintaining integrity, and it is quite another to promote the climate and values that foster individual intellectual honesty and organizational disdain for violating the trust.

The Committee on Science, Engineering, and Public Policy (COSEPUP) of the National Academy of Sciences, the National Academy of Engineering, and the Institute of Medicine has produced a solid framework for *Ensuring the Integrity of the Research Process*. In 12 recommendations, the committee has succinctly stated the responsibilities of individual scientists, research institutions, and government agencies. The committee notes that "the inability of refusal of research institutions to address misconduct-in-science cases can undermine both the integrity of the research process and self governance by the research community."

Every research institution must have a well disseminated policy on scientific misconduct that provides notice of the standards for academic integrity as well as procedures for receiving reports of alleged breaches and the steps for a preliminary inquiry, formal investigation, adjudication, and sanctions. There must be at least one institutional official capable of organizing review and disposition of a case of alleged scientific misconduct, and that individual must be in a position to drop other duties in order to meet the stringent requirements of due process. In "The Laboratory is Not a Courtroom," Charles Maechling, Jr., makes an interesting case for treating such cases in a more "civil law" than "criminal law" manner. He argues that the civil law system offers a model more similar to academic procedures. Regardless, the procedures must be fair and must provide protection of faculty from unwarranted allegations and also provide protection of complainants ("whistleblowers") against reprisals. As a practical matter, if scientific misconduct cases are challenged in a civil or criminal court, the *process used* rather than the *outcome* of the case will be the primary concern. A very useful guide for institutions, *Beyond the Framework,* has recently been developed by the Association of American Medical Colleges. This easy-to-use booklet raises all of the issues that must be considered at every step in the process and offers suggestions on how to proceed.

Of course, the primary institutional effort should be to prevent misconduct through promoting integrity in research. While it is generally recognized that dishonest people will behave dishonestly, it is also clear that students emulate the values of their mentors and role models. Mentoring to promote intellectual honesty is the heart and soul of training scientists. The relationship between student and mentor must be valued as the primary means of inculcating absolute commitment to honesty in the design and performance of experiments and the collection and reporting of results. Institutions must also emphasize the importance of integrity and inculcation of these values in both the MD and PhD curricula. Ed Pellegrino has provided his usual thoughtful and helpful perspectives on the ethical basis of scientific integrity in his chapter *Accountability in Research* ("Character and the Ethical Conduct of Research"). He states, "Those who accept funds for research enter into a covenant with society in which the primary goods cannot be power, personal profit, prestige, or pride . . . Invariably at the foundation of scientific fraud there is an inversion of values and dispositions so that self-interest replaces truth as the ordering principle."

When scientific investigators have a personal financial interest in the outcome of their research, they are considered to have a conflict of interest. There is concern that conflict of interest is a growing threat to scientific integrity. The concern stems from the assumption that scientists should not have opportunities for financial gain if their peers (and others who depend on scientific results) are to believe that their reported results are free of bias. Generally speaking, the concern is with undue bias—not fraud—which is an entirely different matter.

How realistic is it to keep scientists free of outside financial interests? What special problems exist for clinical investigators? How can the university best deal with this problem? What role can industry and government play?

"No conflict—no interest" was the reply given recently by a research administrator when asked to describe his institution's policy on conflict of interest. Although this response may seem glib, it reflects an understanding of the problem and serves as a good starting point for managing conflicts. Research universities must accept their key role in coupling their scientific discoveries with commercial development. It is not sufficient to be tolerant or passively supportive; universities must be proactive. Failure to organize for solid management of the technology transfer process will result in unmanaged conflicts of interest and loss of valuable intellectual property. The federal Technology Transfer Act of 1986 makes it clear that the public expects grantee institutions and their faculty to promote the technology development process.

"No conflict—no interest" reflects the reality that personal and institutional motivational factors for "fame and fortune" are crucial for success. If so, why have some universities and society at large considered pursuit of commercialization to be unacademic? Although the answer to this question is multifaceted, concern for conflict of interest is at the heart of the matter. The motive for substantial financial gain is thought to be too compelling, leading to undue bias in the collection and reporting of research results.

This concern seems greatest for the physician involved in the clinical investigation of medical products. Ironically, the randomized controlled trial (RCT)—the heart of clinical investigation—is unquestionably the most rigorously designed form of scientific research and is subjected to the most scrutiny by committees and government agencies. Certainly the clinical investigator in a multicenter RCT with oversight by a separate data monitoring group has virtually no opportunity to bias the results. In contrast, the bench scientist does not have to contend with any of these external devices.

The basis for the discrepancy relates to concern for the public health implications of the clinical evaluation of medical products. The Food and Drug Administration could not accomplish its regulatory responsibilities if not for complete trust in the results of clinical trials of medical products performed by academic clinical investigators. Shimm and Spece raise concern over the "reimbursement offered to the investigator" for covering the costs of such studies. They are particularly worried when "the reimbursement exceeds the per-patient costs incurred by the investigator."

It is absurd to expect a university to subsidize the Research and Development program of a for-profit company. In effect, the university would be using tuition and/or endowment income to pay for unreimbursed direct costs or overhead. It is unclear what Shimm and Spece mean when they suggest that the "payments . . . go to the medical school dean rather than to the individual investigator." Payments to universities do not go to any individual, dean or investigator, unless they are declared as personal income. Placing the reimbursed costs in a general fund, rather than in the investigator's department or other cost center has the effect of requiring the department to donate the investigator's effort and other costs.

There are many ways for faculty to receive financial benefits, including research grants, consulting fees, royalty and equity (shareholding). Each mode of financial benefit creates a potential for at least the appearance of conflict.

Institutions have primary responsibility for review of cases of conflict of interest and instituting steps that minimize the possibility of undue bias. In cases where the benefits of the conflict are outweighed by the risks to the integrity of the research, the conflict must be eliminated.

Management tools include peer review, public disclosure of the conflict, and escrow of equity until a reasonable time after the completion of the research phase. In order for disclosure of conflicts to be effective, they must be disclosed in each written or oral presentation of scientific results.

If due diligence is undertaken by faculty leaders and by their institutions, it will be possible to restore and maintain the perception and reality of scientific integrity.

CHAPTER VII

Ethical Standards for Scientific Publications

A B S T R A C T S   A N D   E X C E R P T S

■ Bero LA, Galbraith A, Rennie D. The publication of sponsored symposiums in medical journals. *N Engl J Med.* 1992;327:1135-1140.

Abstracted from information appearing in *NEJM*. Reprinted with permission of the *New England Journal of Medicine*.

Background. An increasing proportion of spending by the pharmaceutical industry has gone to funding symposiums that are published by peer-reviewed medical journals. This study tests the hypothesis that such sponsorship, particularly by a single pharmaceutical company, is associated with promotional orientation of the symposium and a distortion of the peer-review process.

Methods. We counted the symposiums published in 58 journals of clinical medicine and surveyed the journal editors regarding their policies for symposium issues. We analyzed the symposium issues that appeared in the 11 journals that published the most symposiums in order to determine the sponsor or sponsors, the topics, whether the titles were misleading, whether brand names were used, and whether the featured drugs were classified by the Food and Drug Administration as innovative or approved.

Results. The number of symposiums published per year increased steadily from 1966 through 1989. Forty-two percent of those analyzed (262 of 625) had a single pharmaceutical company as the sponsor. These symposiums were more likely than those with other sponsors to have misleading titles (P<0.001) and to use brand names (P<0.001), and less likely to be peer-reviewed in the same manner as other articles in the parent journal (P<0.001). Of the 161 symposiums that focused on a single drug, 51 percent concerned unapproved therapies; 14 percent concerned drugs classified as bringing important therapeutic gains.

Conclusions. Symposiums sponsored by drug companies often have promotional attributes and are not peer-reviewed. Financial relations among symposium participants, sponsors, and journals should be completely disclosed, symposiums should be clearly identified, and journal editors should maintain editorial control over contributions from symposiums.

■ **Dickersin K, Min YI, Meinert CL. Factors influencing publication of research results. *JAMA*. 1992;267:374-378.**

Of the studies for which analyses had been reported as having been performed at the time of interview, 81% from the School of Medicine and Hospital and 66% from the School of Hygiene and Public Health had been published. Publication was not associated with sample size, presence of a comparison group, or type of study (eg, observational study vs clinical trial). External funding and multiple data collection sites were positively associated with publication. There was evidence of publication bias in that for both institutional review boards there was an association between results reported to be significant and publication. Contrary to popular opinion, publication bias originates primarily with investigators, not journal editors: only six of the 124 studies not published were reported to have been rejected for publication.

There is a statistically significant association between significant results and publication.

The long-term solution to publication bias lies in systems providing for the registration of studies at the time they are undertaken, prior to the start of data collection. Once established and operational, such systems would provide a means of identification of studies, independent of their publication status.

■ Hillman AL, Eisenberg JM, Pauly MV, et al. Avoiding bias in the conduct and reporting of cost-effectiveness research sponsored by pharmaceutical companies. *N Engl J Med.* 1991;324:1362-1365.

Abstracted from information appearing in *NEJM*. Reprinted with permission of the *New England Journal of Medicine*.

Because of the growing focus on containing health care costs, pharmaceutical companies are trying to demonstrate the cost effectiveness of their products relative to alternatives. In Europe and Australia, economic analyses are often required for government approval and pricing of new pharmaceuticals. In the United States, such analyses are increasingly being used for marketing and to obtain formulary approval. Because of the corporate need for timely results and confidentiality about a new drug in the period before marketing begins and because other financial support is limited, pharmaceutical companies themselves sponsor most academic research into the cost effectiveness of pharmaceuticals. The relationship is symbiotic. Academic researchers—especially young, unestablished investigators—are eager for new sources of funding. At the same time, pharmaceutical marketing benefits from the imprimatur of research published by respected independent academic researchers.

In this article we explore the conduct of industry-sponsored economic analysis. We offer examples of some specific biases that may occur because of the behavior of the investigator, the sponsoring company, or both. We explore whether there is a role for regulation by the Food and Drug Administration. Finally, we offer suggestions for structuring the relationship between industry and academia so that bias is minimized in economic analyses of pharmaceuticals.

We offer the following eight recommendations.

First, written agreements between pharmaceutical companies and investigators should be in the form of research grants to universities, rather than contracts with individual investigators or universities.

Second, economic analyses are by their nature comparative. The selection of alternatives to be compared should be based on their clinical relevance, not on the potential favorability of the results.

Third, investigators should be allowed to expand the company's study design to include additional types of costs, economic perspectives, and comparison drugs as data permit.

Fourth, if projects are funded in a series of steps rather than by one large grant, results should not be provided to be the sponsor until publication is guaranteed and funded.

Fifth, investigators should be vigilant to the temptation to produce favorable findings.

Sixth, investigators should publish valid results regardless of their promotional value to the sponsoring company, and journal editors should try to avoid a bias against publishing negative results.

Finally, researchers should take all reasonable steps to ensure that the level of funding permits methodologically sound, clinically relevant results with enough statistical power to detect important differences among the alternatives compared.

■ **Koren G, Klein N. Bias against negative studies in newspaper reports of medical research. *JAMA*. 1991;266:1824-1826.**

Objective.—To assess if the reporting of controversial medical journal articles by newspapers reflects the existence of a bias against negative studies (those showing no effect), we compared the rates of newspaper reporting of two studies, one negative and one positive, published back-to-back in the March 20, 1991, issue of *JAMA*. Both studies analyzed an area of public health concern, radiation as a risk for cancer.

Design.—Seven computerized on-line databases were screened for daily newspapers published in North America during the week following *JAMA*'s publication of the two studies. These databases had full-text access to 168 daily newspapers. Newspapers identified with reports of the two studies were analyzed for length and quality of the reports.

Results.—Seventeen newspapers, publishing 19 reports on the two studies, were identified. Nine reports were dedicated solely to the positive study and 10 reports covered both studies. None of the reports were dedicated to the negative study only. In reports covering both studies, the mean length of the positive reports was significantly longer than the mean length of the negative reports. The mean quality score of the positive reports was significantly higher than that of the negative reports.

Conclusions.—The number, length, and quality of newspaper reports on the positive study were greater than news reports on the negative study, which suggests a bias against news reports of studies showing no effects or no adverse effects.

The well-known media phrase that "good news is no news" may be detrimental in the biomedical context, as it helps perpetuate a bias against negative studies. Responsible journalists should acknowledge the importance of providing balanced information to the public when covering controversial health issues and should give equal attention to positive and negative studies.

■ Rennie D, Flanagin A, Glass RM. Conflicts of interest in the publication of science. *JAMA*. 1991;266:266-267.

Editors, too, should be alert to conflicts of interest in the authorship, review, rejection, and acceptance of manuscripts. Last year a congressional subcommittee assigned to investigate scientific misconduct determined that biomedical journals have led the academic community by ensuring proper disclosure of conflicts of interest even though their options to do so are limited. Editors have generally agreed that financial conflicts of interest may not necessarily bias the author or invalidate a study, and many editors believe that disclosure to the reader is an appropriate way to deal with such conflict.

Although journal requirements to disclose conflicts of interest have been routine for a number of years, such requirements still seem new and unfamiliar to many authors.

Editors are not and should not be the science police. We do not believe that authors' financial interests automatically invalidate the results of their investigations or that reviewers' conflicts invalidate their criticisms of manuscripts. We do believe, however, that editors should not have financial conflicts of interest. We also believe that it is the editors' responsibility to ensure that authors and reviewers disclose all potential conflicts of interest when submitting their manuscripts or reviews, and we will continue to rely on the integrity of authors and reviewers to comply with our requests for such disclosure.

■ Safer DJ, Krager JM. Effect of a media blitz and a threatened lawsuit on stimulant treatment. *JAMA*. 1992;268:1004-1007.

Objective.—To enumerate and evaluate changes in the rate of medication treatment for hyperactive/inattentive students subsequent to negative media publicity about methylphenidate (Ritalin) and related lawsuits threatened or initiated from late 1987 to early 1989.

Design.—Biennial 1971 to 1991 school nurse surveys of medication treatment for hyperactive/inattentive students; a 1989 school nurse questionnaire on parent attitudes about medication; annual 1984 through 1991 hyperkinetic clinic treatment data; annual 1986 through 1990 Drug Enforcement Administration estimates of retail sales of methylphenidate, nationally and locally.

Primary Setting.—All public and private elementary and secondary schools in

Baltimore County, Maryland.

Patients.—Students receiving medication for hyperactivity/inattentiveness.

Results.—Whereas the medication rate for the treatment of hyperactive/inattentive students in Baltimore County doubled every 4 to 7 years from 1971 through 1987, it declined 39% in the 1989 and 1991 surveys from its 1987 peak. This drop occurred after the 1987 through 1989 media blitz against methylphenidate and after a well-publicized threatened lawsuit locally. Parents became fearful of media-reported medication "side effects" and school staff hesitated to refer restless, impulsive, and inattentive students to physicians. Most inhibited from the prospect of medication treatment were less affluent parents and parents of hyperactive/inattentive elementary school children who had never received medication. Drug Enforcement Administration data revealed that the Baltimore metropolitan area had a far greater decline in methylphenidate use than that which occurred nationally.

Conclusion.—Strong circumstantial evidence suggests that the prominent 1989 and 1991 declines in the initiation of stimulant medication for hyperactive/inattentive students were related to the apprehension of parents and involved professionals generated by the methylphenidate media blitz and the threatened lawsuit.

■ **Wilkes MS, Doblin BH, Shapiro MF. Pharmaceutical advertisements in leading medical journals: experts' assessments.** *Annals of Internal Medicine.* **1992;116:912-919.**

Reprinted with permission of the *Annals of Internal Medicine.*

Objective: To assess both the accuracy of scientific data presented in print pharmaceutical advertisements and the compliance of these advertisements with current Food and Drug Administration (FDA) standards.

Design: Cross-sectional survey.

Measurements: Each full-page pharmaceutical advertisement (n=109) appearing in 10 leading medical journals, along with all available references cited in the advertisement (82% of the references cited were available) were sent to three reviewers: two physicians in the relevant clinical area who were experienced in peer review and one academic clinical pharmacist. Reviewers, 95% of whom responded, were asked to evaluate the advertisements using criteria based on FDA guidelines, to judge the educational value and overall quality of the advertisements, and to make a recommendation regarding publication.

Results: In 30% of cases, two or more reviewers disagreed with the advertisers' claim that the drug was the "drug of choice." Reviewers felt that information on efficacy was balanced with that on side effects and contraindications in 49% of advertisements but was not balanced in 40%. Reviewers agreed with advertisements' claims that the drug was safe in 86% of the cases but judged that headlines in 32% of the advertisements containing headlines misled the reader about efficacy. In 44% of cases, reviewers felt that the advertisement would lead to improper prescribing if a physician had no other information about the drug other than that contained in the advertisement. Fifty-seven percent of advertisements were judged by two or more reviewers to have little or no educational value. Overall, reviewers would not have recommended publication of 28% of the advertisements and would have required major revisions in 34% before publication.

Conclusion: In the opinion of the reviewers, many advertisements contained deficiencies in areas in which the FDA has established explicit standards of quality. New strategies are needed to ensure that advertisements comply with standards intended to promote proper use of the products and to protect the consumer.

COMMENTARY
James E. Dalen

Although directed to physicians and medical scientists, medical journals have a very real impact on the public at large. Therefore, examination of the ethical standards of these scientific publications is an appropriate public concern.

The most important issue is what information gets published in medical journals! Dickersin and his colleagues examined research studies performed at Johns Hopkins to see which were eventually published in medical journals. The vast majority (more than 66 percent) of studies resulted in publication. Studies least likely to be published were those that the investigators judged to have results that were not significant. Only six of 124 studies that were not published were submitted to, and rejected by, a medical journal. Thus, the obvious first gatekeepers to determine what gets published are the investigators themselves.

Once an article is submitted for publication, the next gatekeepers are the thousands of peer-reviewers who serve without pay and usually without recognition. Editors and editorial boards rely heavily on these reviewers who are selected for their expertise in the subject of the investigation.

Rennie and his colleagues discuss how conflicts of interest could influence these two groups of gatekeepers—the authors and the reviewers. Financial conflicts of interest could motivate authors and/or reviewers. They may have financial interests that would be affected by the publication of positive or negative information about a particular product or device. In response to this concern, authors, peer reviewers, and even editorial boards and editors are often asked to sign a financial disclosure form to identify any potential conflict of interest. Data as to the effectiveness of these disclosure forms are lacking.

The Rennie article points out that "intellectual" conflicts of interest are another potential determinant of what does and what does not get published in our medical journals. Are peer reviewers likely to be receptive to manuscripts that disagree with either the published data of reviewers or unpublished views of the subject at hand? It should be clear that editors cannot determine if the submission and reviews of investigations have been influenced by conflict of interest by the authors or the reviewers. Written disclosures of potential conflicts of interest are useful in reminding authors and reviewers of this issue. However, in the final analysis, the editor and the readers must depend upon the integrity of the authors and the reviewers.

Another force in determining what gets published in medical journals is the pharmaceutical industry. Most medical journals rely heavily on income derived from pharmaceutical advertising. Without this income, some journals could not survive and, therefore, would not be published.

Many physicians believe that they are not influenced by the ads. Yet, the pharmaceutical industry spends hundreds of millions of dollars per year in the belief that these ads do affect physicians and their prescription writing. These ads must comply with requirements of the Food and Drug Administration (FDA) as to their accuracy. Wilkes and his colleagues present data to indicate that many of these ads do not comply with the FDA requirements for accuracy. It would appear that the FDA may lack the resources to ensure compliance with its standards for accuracy. The FDA suggestions that medical journals play a larger role in ensuring the accuracy of pharmaceutical advertising are unlikely to be accepted by these medical journals.

In addition to determining what advertising get published, pharmaceutical companies have an impact on what specific studies are published in medical journals. In the most extreme case, an entire issue or supplement of a medical journal may be devoted to the publication of a symposium sponsored by a pharmaceutical company. Bero, Galbraith, and Rennie reviewed the publication of such symposia by 58 journals of clinical medicine and found that the number of such symposia increased each year from 1966 to 1989.

They noted that some symposia, sponsored by drug companies, have promotional attributes and are not peer reviewed. The Bero article recommends guidelines for such symposia that would enhance the appropriateness of these publications. Nearly all of these symposia include a guest editor. The guest editor bears particular responsibility for ensuring that these publications are peer reviewed and balanced.

By sponsoring specific research projects, drug companies (and other major funding agencies such as the National Institutes of Health) have a major impact on what studies are performed and, therefore, are subsequently submitted for publication. It is standard practice to acknowledge drug company sponsorship when manuscripts are submitted for review. Reviewers' decisions may or may not be influenced by noting drug company sponsorship.

Drug companies also sponsor studies of the cost-effectiveness of various products. Hillman and his colleagues reported that this can lead to some special problems. Research-oriented personnel rather than marketing departments of pharmaceutical companies usually oversee these studies. The potential effect of economic findings on sales volumes may lead to difficult issues of conflict of interest.

What gets published in medical journals is determined by the interactions of authors, peer reviewers, editorial boards, editors, the pharmaceutical industry, and other agencies that sponsor research.

The end product—the journal with its scientific reports and its advertising—obviously directly impacts physicians. To the extent that it influences their practice patterns, it affects their patients and the public. Medical journals have a direct impact on the public via the press in addition to the indirect effect caused by influencing the practice patterns of physicians.

For many people, newspaper accounts of what appears in medical journals may be their primary source of medical information. Some medical journals encourage the press to report on certain of their articles by producing press releases for the lay press. However, it is up to the press to decide which articles to report, and how to report them. Koren and Klein studied how the press reported two back-to-back articles on radiation as a risk factor for cancer that appeared in the *Journal of the American Medical Association*. The authors found that more newspapers reported the study that suggested that radiation is a significant risk factor for cancer than the accompanying article that found no significant risk. The number, length, and quality of the newspaper accounts of the study showing that radiation is a risk factor for cancer greatly exceeded the newspaper accounts of the negative report. By deciding which articles to report, and how to report them, the lay press determines what the public should know about current medical research.

It is a long trail from the inception to completion of research studies and then to submission to and publication by medical journals and finally to reports in the lay press. It is a potentially hazardous trail; potential conflicts of interest may appear at many points in the trail. A safe journey depends upon the integrity of investigators, reviewers, editorial boards, the pharmaceutical industry, other sponsoring agencies, editors, and the lay press.

COMMENTARY

H. Garland Hershey, Jr.

This set of articles focuses primarily on two potential threats to the maintenance of high ethical standards for scientific publications: conflict of interest and biased reporting. These two problem areas and other threats such as fraud, plagiarism, submission of manuscripts to more than one journal, and irresponsible coauthorship raise several questions in the mind of a concerned reader. Perhaps the first question is, "What effect has peer review in protecting the integrity of scientific publications?" For all its considerable value in promoting the quality of journal articles, peer review should not be expected to guard against threats to ethical standards in publishing as Relman and Angell note in their 1989

New England Journal of Medicine editorial on this topic. "Peer-review is not and cannot be an objective scientific process, nor can it be relied upon to guarantee the validity or honesty of scientific research," according to these authors. Maintenance of high standards in health publications, then, is the province not of a process like peer review, but of actions by authors, editors, funding agencies, government, and most important for our purposes, leaders of academic health centers.

The fact that peer review cannot be relied on to protect against ethical breeches is illustrated clearly in the article by Bero, Galbraith, and Rennie. These authors describe how conflict of interest can subvert the peer review process and demonstrate that symposia sponsored by pharmaceutical companies and published in peer-reviewed journals often have misleading titles, mention brand names, and "are less likely to be peer-reviewed in the same manner as other articles in the parent journal." In fact these articles may not be peer reviewed at all. The result is that readers may get inaccurate impressions about the use and value of medications. Consequently, as the authors note, publication of drug company sponsored symposia in the peer-reviewed scientific literature conceivably "can influence the prescribing practices of physicians." Perhaps this explains why the pharmaceutical industry spent $88 million on symposia in 1988 (up from $6 million in 1975).

Although Bero, Galbraith, and Rennie focus on symposia sponsored by drug companies, there is no reason to expect that similar symposia funded by other companies with vested interests in selling their products do not also subvert the peer-review process to their advantage. What can be done to counter this threat to the ethical conduct of scientific publishing? The authors suggest that several players—government, journal editors, publishers, drug companies, symposium speakers, journal readers, and importantly, universities—have roles to play. The role for leaders of academic health centers is ". . . to maintain complete control over the selection of the topic, the speakers, and any articles to be published" as a result of symposia, which are co-sponsored by more than one company. This can reduce promotional bias. This is excellent advice for dealing with an increasingly common and powerful manipulation of scientific publishing by any funding agency, whether or not it is a drug company, that is susceptible to conflict of interest between objective reporting and product promotion.

It is disappointing, but perhaps not surprising, that conflict of interest also appears to affect the accuracy of information presented in pharmaceutical advertisements in health science journals. Wilkes, Doblin, and Shapiro found that large numbers of drug advertisements in leading journals do not meet the standards for quality of the Food and Drug Administration. As the authors point out, peer-reviewed "medical journals derive substantial income from advertisements" for drugs. Thus "the pharmaceutical industry has the potential to exert enormous influence over (these) journals." In an era of growing competition, journal editors could be torn between accepting accurate advertisement and gaining important advertising revenue. The potential for conflict of interest to affect the content of information on virtually every page—advertisements as well as articles—in scientific publications is very real.

Pharmaceutical companies are also targeted in the article by Hillman and his colleagues. In this instance, the conflict is between the conduct of scientifically sound research and promotion of drugs. Those in a position of conflict are researchers who are funded by pharmaceutical companies to conduct economic analyses of drugs produced by those companies. The authors suggest that the "companies consider economic analyses to be marketing devices more than scientific or clinical research." Here, again, leaders of academic health centers can have a positive influence by ensuring that this kind of research is funded by grants rather than contracts as is often done, along with requiring that publication of the research results remain the sole province of the researcher. Clearly, these are not foolproof safeguards, but they are basic principles that can reduce the incidence of adverse effects of conflict of interest.

Bias in the reporting of research findings is not generated by conflict of interest alone. Dickersin, Min, and Meinert, for example, conclude that researchers tend not to submit articles without significant findings, and Koren and Klein describe a study indicating that newspapers are biased against reporting studies that show no positive effects. Safer and Krager illustrate the power of the media to influence behavior in their account of the widespread negative publicity about Ritalin and its apparent impact on the marked reduction in the use of the drug for treating hyperactivity and inattentiveness among students in the schools in Baltimore County, Maryland. According to the article, the "media blitz was spearheaded by the major national television talk show hosts. . . who allowed anecdotal and unsubstantiated critical allegations concerning Ritalin use and [its] side effects to be aired." Peer review may be imperfect, but it helps to assure quality in scientific publishing. It is also an important safeguard against the indiscriminate dissemination of scientific information, which may be erroneous or dangerous and has the potential to influence the health-related behaviors of practitioners and patients alike.

Rennie, Flanagin, and Glass correctly note that conflicts of interest may not necessarily bias authors or invalidate studies. But as several of these articles suggest, conflict of interest can and does create bias. And when the media widely disseminate information, as noted in several articles, information can profoundly influence behavior. The related issues of conflict and bias are significant and can have significant consequences. Rennie, Flanagin, and Glass believe that journal "editors should not be the science police." Neither should leaders of academic health centers, nor researchers, funding agencies, government regulators, and users of scientific information. But all groups have a role in upholding ethical standards for scientific publications.

It is important for each of these groups to understand their roles and responsibilities. For leaders of academic health centers, responsibilities include promoting an atmosphere of openness and trust rather than secrecy and suspicion among faculty and students. Leaders have responsibilities to promote effective mentoring of junior faculty by senior faculty, and deal with possible cases of misconduct promptly, objectively, and carefully. These actions are reasonable to protect both the accuser and the accused during the course of the inquiry. These responsibilities also include setting and enforcing policies like those suggested above to minimize the likelihood of conflict of interest and bias in the conduct of research and the dissemination of research findings. The role of the leaders of academic health centers in dealing with these issues is not easy, but it is essential if we are to responsibly discharge our role as stewards of the scientific process, our fellow scientists and health care providers, and our patients.

CHAPTER VIII

Public Perceptions of Science: Dilemmas for Policymaking

ABSTRACTS AND EXCERPTS

■ **Institute of Medicine. *Biomedical Politics*. Hanna KE, ed. Washington, D.C.: National Academy Press, 1991.**

The decision-making process [in biomedical research] is the focus of this report. Examining the way discourse proceeds among all affected parties in a policy debate may shed light on how the decision was made and could provide clues as to how similar decisions might best be debated in the future. It is not the purpose of this effort to judge whether the decisions described in the following cases were proper or improper. Rather, the goal is better understanding so that appropriate questions may be asked in the future when difficult decisions must be made.

The historical case study was chosen as the methodology for this effort, with the cases serving as prototypes for appropriate or inappropriate strategies for decision making.

The cases were selected based on a set of criteria that constitute characteristic facets of a biomedical policy problem. . . . as a set they illustrate the texture of decision making in the field of health sciences research.

. . . the first case . . . reports on the activities that led to the 1989 Food and Drug Administration decision to approve the use of dideoxyinosine (ddI), an as yet unproven AIDS therapy in a parallel track protocol.

. . . the second case . . . provides an overview of action and inaction in the heated debate over the inavailability of RU-486 (the "French abortion pill") in the United States.

. . . the third case . . . chronicles the events of 1986-1990 leading to congressional action on the human genome project.

The fourth case . . . analyzes the events leading to the passage of Section 299I of the Social Security Amendments of 1972, which produced an entitlement program for victims of end-stage renal disease.

. . . case five . . . describes the deliberations of the Human Fetal Tissue Transplantation Research panel in its efforts to provide advice to the Department of Health and Human Services on the morality of using fetal tissue obtained from induced abortions for therapeutic transplantation.

. . . the last case . . . takes us back to the 1970s and describes the events that led to and included the Asilomar conference on recombinant deoxyribonucleic acid (DNA).

These cases illustrate the complexity and evolution of decision making related to the diffusion and adoption of advances in biomedicine. The committee did not judge whether the cases were resolved adequately; in fact, in many of these cases the debate is still in process. What makes this collection different from other "technology transfer" reports is the deliberate intent to include the impact of values and the role of the public in the discussion. The cases do not merely present a historical, descriptive documentation of the diffusion process. Integral to the final analyses is a discussion of the myriad moral, religious, political, legal, psychological, and economic forces that influence how and when certain decisions are made.

■ **Jasanoff S. Does public understanding influence public policy?** *Chemistry & Industry.* **1991;15:537-540.**

Reprinted with permission of the Society of Chemical Industry.

Two decades of intense public preoccupation with chemicals have laid the groundwork for assessing how the public perceives science, why science often lends itself to contradictory perceptions, and how elements of the public understanding of science can be put to work to produce better and more rational regulatory policies.

Some recent events shed light on the wellsprings of public concern over chemicals, and in each case, some of the structural features of modern science and technology have exacerbated rather than dampened risk-averse reactions from the public. These examples are drawn chiefly from the US, where connections between public understanding and public policy are unusually direct and transparent. The lessons and implications of these cases, however, can be generalized beyond the political boundaries of the US, because they relate to universal characteristics of scientific knowledge and its technological uses.

Examples like the dioxin and *Alar* controversies can be multiplied many times over, but they all point to certain recurrent sources of public disaffection. The first of these is the extent and quality of public participation in key aspects of chemical policymaking.

A second major source of conflict between the chemical industry and the public concerns the appropriate role of science and scientists in determining policies for technology.

. . . when science is conducted to serve policy objectives it invariably becomes entwined with social considerations. Policy-relevant science is produced under extraordinary constraints of time, money, and politics, and it is routinely confronted with problems that defy theoretical and methodological consensus-building. As a result, the findings of such science are more obviously negotiated, convention-bound, and value-laden than are the typical findings of academic scientific research.

The third source of concern is the relationship of scientific change to policy change. Among the most serious difficulties in making policy for science and technology is that the two major participants — scientists and policy -makers — are driven by two very different kinds of rationality.

Examining the basis for public fears about chemical risk expands our own understanding of science, illuminating the complex ways in which factually uncertain knowledge interacts with the social organisation and institutional control of scientific activity. This expanded understanding in turn should promote the design of more effective institutions and processes for public policy.

■ **Silverstone R. Communicating science to the public. *Science, Technology, & Human Values.* 1991;16:106-110.**

One set of projects in the U.K. research program on public understanding of science explored three areas in which science is on the communication agenda: in the mass media, in the museum, and in the school.

The projects share, with different degrees of emphasis, four main assumptions, supported by the literature.

1. There is no such thing as *the* communication of science. Neither science nor the media environment is a unified phenomenon.

2. There is no such thing as *the* public. There are many publics for science.

3. In the modern communication environment, science cannot claim any privileged status. Science has to compete for attention, from the producers and the receivers of communication.

4. The omnipresence of the media does not equal omnipotence.

Four broad themes are emerging from the communication projects, all of which are still in progress.

The communication of science is complex phenomenon, affected by a range of institutional imperatives and constraints, which influence not just *how much* science is communicated but also the nature of that science.

Science is never communicated in a vacuum. The institutional environments of communication provide a powerful mediation of their own.

Science is constructed, therefore, not only in the production of science communications—in the programs, articles, galleries, or lessons in which science is the subject. Science is also constructed—perhaps reconstructed is a better way of putting it—by the viewers, readers, visitors, and pupils, who receive the communications.

Much of the preceding has pointed to constraints: of national culture, organizational structure, practicalities of work in the media or the museum, local knowledges, interests, skills, and expertise of those who both produce and receive communications. A final constraint is the wider political and economic environment. Government decisions on museum charges, broadcasting policies, and the national curriculum will all affect not just the quantity but also the quality, not just the forms but also the content, of public understanding of science.

■ **Veatch RM. Consensus of expertise: the role of consensus of experts in formulating public policy and estimating facts.** *J Med Philos.* **1991;16:427-445.**

Reprinted with permission of Kluwer Academic Publishers.

For years analysts have recognized the error of assuming that experts in medical science are also experts in deciding the clinically correct course for patients. This paper extends the analysis of the use of the consensus of experts to their use in public policy groups such as NIH Consensus Development panels. After arguing that technical experts cannot be expected to be expert on public policy decisions, the author extends the criticism to the use of the consensus of experts in estimating facts to provide a basis for policy decisions. It is argued that to the extent that (a) experts' views regarding a body of facts can be expected to correlate with their values relevant to those facts; and (b) the values of experts differ from the values of lay people, even the estimates of the facts given by the consensus of expert panels can be expected to differ from the estimates lay people would have given had they had the relevant scientific expertise.

. . . the implications for the use of panels of experts in the public policy process are radical. Even for the admittedly impossible task for providing unbiased estimates of facts upon which policy makers might later act the answers given by panels of experts ought to reflect their consensus values and their consensus values ought to be different from those of the general public. Caution seems to be in order. Some strategies might be available for attempting to adjust for this seemingly necessary distortion.

One plausible strategy would be to arrange for multiple panels purposely structured based on the values of the experts constituting them.

Another strategy might be to stratify the sampling of experts so that it reflects the value distribution of the general public rather than the value distribution of the experts.

Still another possibility is letting the consensus panels work as they have in the past generating consensuses about more factual questions, but recognizing that the their [sic] report ought to be distorted somewhat in the direction of the value consensus of the expert group and then making a political adjustment of the estimate of the facts to correct for this distortion.

■ **Wynne B. Knowledges in context.** *Science, Technology, & Human Values.* **1991;16:111-121.**

Our projects begin by exploring the relationships between "citizens" and "sources" —between members and groups of the public and that diverse body of institutions, knowledges, and disciplinary specialists that we term *science.*

. . . studying the public understanding of science requires us to devote equal attention to the various ways scientists themselves understand, interpret, and represent "science." Otherwise, we tacitly consolidate the false view that the problems all have to do with the public's understandings rather than also with scientists and scientific institutions.

. . . in everyday life people have to interpret and negotiate scientific knowledge in conjunction with other forms of knowledge. We have also stressed the fact that science is itself far from unproblematic but is instead often partial, temporally contingent, conflicting, and uncertain to a degree that public statements rarely acknowledge.

. . . to advance public understanding of science we need to encourage more awareness and debate about the institutional forms in which scientific knowledge is both presented and created. Our research shows people to be astute at taking up science as a *means* (when the right social conditions prevail) but wary about its *ends* and *interests*. Thus enhancement of public uptake of science would appear to require the development of multiple institutional forms of science, with correspondingly diverse audiences, patrons, interests, and objectives. This would also meet the need for more diverse, independent, and context-sensitive sources of scientific information.

However, we need to be aware that the *overall* trend in the structure and control of science is currently running in the opposite direction to the one indicated here. Indeed, it is worth asking whether the current concern about the public understanding of science does not reflect a deeper anxiety about the further intensification of the centralized ownership and control of science as a private resource rather than a public good. While many commentators portray a lack of public understanding of science as an obstacle to democratic vitality, it may be that the reverse is also true; that impoverished democracy and intensifying hegemony around science is a major obstacle to the enhanced public understanding of science.

■ Wynne B. Public perception and communication of risks: what do we know? *The Journal of NIH Research.* 1991;3:65-70.

Reprinted with permission from *The Journal of NIH Research.*

The study of public perceptions of risks and public understanding of science has become a growing research field that combines the social and natural sciences. Some well-grounded and widely accepted insights have emerged. These have important implications for the ways that scientists represent themselves in public, but also for the institutional structures by which science and technology are managed.

Risk-perception research has made inroads into explaining the frustrating dynamics of such risk debates. . . . Social science research has identified various objective "attributes" of risks, such as reversibility, voluntariness, familiarity, and concentration of damage.

One of the most pervasive dimensions of risk situations that logically affects public perceptions and responses is the trustworthiness of the agent(s) in control of the risks.

. . . expert institutions are also influenced by their cultural and institutional context in the way they interpret technical uncertainties and define technical risks.

Risks are mediated by the social institutions that create and control them. These institutions represent risks to various publics, but they also directly affect the magnitudes of the risks, depending on the diligence with which they control them.

The very development and not just the application of scientific knowledge is increasingly tied to policy situations in which incomplete knowledge is pressed into policy use and developed in the public setting, not in professional seclusion.

A more resilient and mature policy process—one in which both the scientists and the public are capable of authentic learning—would recognize in principle these social dimensions of risk assessment, and would seek the institutional mechanisms for constructive negotiation based on different kinds of knowledge and experience.

■ Ziman J. Public understanding of science. *Science, Technology, & Human Values.* 1991;16:99-105.

Concern about the gap between the world of science and the world at large is nothing new. The British Association and other similar bodies were founded in the early nineteenth century to fill this gap.

Nevertheless, there has long been a feeling that these efforts were not having much effect. It seemed a paradox that so many people should have so little understanding of the science that dominates their culture.

These concerns came to a head in the report of the Royal Society Committee chaired by Dr. (now Sir) Walter Bodmer, which appeared in 1985.

. . . it was surprising to us how very little serious research had been done on the subject. . . . Thus the plan for a major program of research to follow up on the Bodmer Report was widely welcomed.

Overall, the most important finding of the research program is that "science" is not a well-bounded, coherent thing, capable of being more or less "understood." This finding is not in any sense a subversive attack on the marvelous and immense body of knowledge produced by scientists, engineers, physicians, technologists, and other researchers. Instead, it is a reminder that what counts as science is sometimes defined very differently by different people—or even by the same people under different circumstances.

The results coming out of the various projects . . . are beginning to jell around a few broad principles:

Incoherence. People do not draw on stable, if fragmented or ill-conceived, "models" of the world, along the lines of textbook accounts of scientific knowledge.

Inadequacy. The use that people make of formal knowledge in any particular situation depends on the needs of the moment and represents only one element in a complex and varied response.

Incredibility. People do not accept passively the knowledge presented to them by scientific "experts."

Inconsistency. Public conflicts on social issues between scientific experts inevitably downgrade the privileged position of scientific knowledge.

COMMENTARY

Herbert Pardes

In organizing this commentary I have tried to emphasize major parts of the articles included in this chapter. I have not worried about comprehensiveness, but rather I have tried to highlight particularly salient and/or useful points. The public has become increasingly involved in scientific policy issues. News is quickly dispensed on diverse issues, and science news is now of interest to an enlarged segment of society due perhaps to the extraordinary information explosion in the last two decades. In the past, scientific opinion was generally accepted as the authoritative statement on a scientific issue. There is now much greater room for question, challenge, difference of opinion, and outright reversal of policy positions advocated by the scientists themselves.

As a result, the notion that consistency, predictability, and rationality may characterize the decision-making process and the final policy outcome may be wishful thinking. Political influences, issues of personality, and simply fortuitous events can be critical in determining the way a policy question will be resolved. Important trends that are bringing about public involvement in policy are a result of increased participation by various segments of society in shaping social directions, including the civil rights and women's movements, as well as current public interest in environmental issues. These forces can profoundly influence science policy decision making.

This wider involvement in decision making induces more inquiry regarding how policy is made and who is involved in resolving policy questions. Increasingly, one sees consumers and citizens on review groups, which previously comprised only professionals. To involve larger segments of society may dilute positions, but it usually increases the likelihood of broader endorsement of whatever consensus position is ultimately realized.

One can convene panels to get comprehensive views. If policy panels do not have authority, they will often be more aggressive and courageous in making suggestions which those decision makers in positions of responsibility may have to reject.

Also, increasingly there are situations in which there are frank disagreements, such as issues related to abortion or RU 486. In those instances, resolution often requires interpersonal mediation and negotiation. If there is simply frank and irreconcilable conflict, whoever has the greater authority or power may decide policy.

It is noteworthy that decision making with regard to policy often can be heavily influenced by one or two people or by a small dedicated group. For the most part, large segments of a society are unconcerned about general policy issues, and yet a determined few can make or press an issue well beyond the range that their limited numbers would imply. It has been said that it takes about eight telephone calls to get a congressperson's attention.

Single-issue groups, such as the anti-abortion or animal rights activists, can obstruct or prevent valuable scientific enterprises. It is also noteworthy that not everybody plays by the rules. The capacity of "single-issue people" to distort is great. Further, when people are sufficiently impassioned about an issue, the means of advocacy may become inconsequential.

In assessing the public role, one has to realize that the vast variation in educational status may leave some individuals with distorted or impoverished capacity to understand science, as Dr. Wynne points out. Also, some segments of the public may expect no risk in a scientific development. This is an important reminder of the formidable nature of public expectations of science. It is also noteworthy, according to Dr. Jasanoff, that once an idea enters the public consciousness, it is difficult to modify.

Generally it is assumed that increased scientific education or understanding will usually bring positive results. While there is probably a correlation between the two, the extent of the correlation is probably less than many would like. Dr. Jasanoff notes that the public may confuse small and large risks. She points out that people will drive with abandon at 80 miles an hour and yet pale at the thought of trace amounts of dioxin.

Aside from the ostensible value of the public understanding science, there also seems to be a correlation between knowing about science and being interested in science. Which factor arises first may be open to question. Ziman makes an important distinction between the value of understanding and specific attitudes in science. Understanding of science is associated with support for obviously useful science. In contrast, the opposite may happen with science that is contentious morally. By educating the public with regard to morally contentious issues, one might find more opposition to the research.

Ziman's studies that analyze the factors that correlate with general interest in science may provide useful information for determining policies for how to educate and inform people about science.

Another very important participant in policy is the press. Often the definition of a problem by the press sets the entire agenda and tone of the discussion of policy. Such a situation argues the need for involving the press early on in scientific projects and for continued contact and education of the press by professionals and scientists.

Different kinds of press complicate the process of disseminating information regarding science. The general press reports with different emphasis than the specialized scientific press. Also, news stories that describe science in the context of scientific discoveries, as opposed to those that frame science in relation to social issues, are appreciated in totally different ways. One finds a kind of positive and proactive statement in the former and often acrimony and conflict in the latter.

It is distressing that in most surveys of the public the level of scientific knowledge is low. Ziman highlights the responsibility of institutions and concerned professionals to improve the transfer process of knowledge into various elements of society, including the schools and the media.

Given the formidable nature of reaching positive policy developments, it is important also that scientists reach agreement as much as possible among themselves. Disagreement between scientists on either budgetary or policy issues often is dangerous or even perhaps fatal for a preferred position. As soon as the professional community splits on an issue, one can assume there will be citizens supporting both sides of the issue. Jasanoff speaks eloquently of the role of expert panels and "getting the science right" in this regard.

I would go further and say that probably the best chance for positive policy or positive budgetary support for science results from collaboration between professional and citizen groups. A combined message usually is particularly impressive to representatives of the legislative or executive branches of government.

Important in enhancing public understanding of science is the need for scientists to speak in terms that are understandable to everyone. At one point, Congressman George E. Brown (D-Ca.) complained that scientists had to give up their right to speak incomprehensively. Ziman also points out the importance of clear and understandable presentations. But, of course, the capacity for the understanding of science varies. Aside from the differences in audience, we have to recognize, as Ziman points out, that what counts in science is often defined differently by different people. Dr. Silverstone also highlights the variability in important aspects of science policy. He states there is no such thing as "the communication" of science, no such thing as "the public," and no privileged status for science. He also highlights the heterogenous nature of the media.

Most of the writers on scientific policy making and public perception stress the importance of the context for any public policy position. It is noteworthy, as Dr. Wynne notes, that survey results can show science generally being held in high esteem, but on a specific issue science is viewed as apathetic and obstructionist. One has but to look at the problems of the University of California, San Francisco School of Medicine, which has been having difficulty developing more in the way of a scientific enterprise, by virtue of concerns among the relatively sophisticated public regarding what that science will be.

Dr. Wynne states that the treatment of uncertainties regarding some scientific or technical issue reflects the political culture. He notes that a technical risk may be seen as a higher risk by regulatory bodies in the United States than in the United Kingdom. This is a graphic reflection of the effect of different contexts in different countries.

Many other issues influence attitudes regarding science, including parental attitudes towards science, as well as attitudes of friends towards schools, youth culture, and achievement. These have substantial impact in determining attitudes towards science. Diverse sorts of studies confirm that science is perceived personally.

To usefully study policy making and public perceptions of science, it is important to realize how diverse a population may be and what baggage people may bring to any scientific issues. Public understanding, as Dr. Wynne points out, is very much an interactive process rather than a simple statement from professional to public that receives automatic acceptance. Dr. Wynne's emphasis on providing "flexible social access to diverse sources of scientific information" is well advised over the notion of giving one simple explanation of the scientific policy.

To summarize: The public is far more involved of late in policy making. The public's attitude towards science and the making of science policy is highly complicated and varied. Public attitudes vary with political and cultural contexts, with the nature of the audience, and with the degree of agreement in the scientific community. The public's stance on science policy issues is very much dependent on fortuitous, political, and personal events.

Science for scientists is an important and serious social venture. They prefer science policy to be rational in content as well as rational in the way the policy is determined. It is distressing to many scientists that cherished principles that determine their function can be subject to randomness and whim.

Perhaps, the most important message is for those such as scientists who are set upon developing socially valuable science policy. They must recognize the need, in informing people about science and bringing about technology transfer, to be alert to these considerably diverse threads in order to have the most receptive and unbiased audience for science and to insure that the science is facilitated rather than obstructed.

COMMENTARY

William A. Peck

We live amid an explosion of public awareness, scrutiny, and criticism. No institution, program, or process is spared. Increasingly sophisticated media methods bombard the public with a seemingly inexhaustible stream of real time or recently generated news, investigative reports, and editorials. Adding to society's impatience and litigiousness is an unprecedented degree of lability, factionalism, and loss of perspective. Hence several reported instances of research fraud, among thousands of research projects, taint all of science. And decisionmakers react.

Polls and other vehicles provide decisionmakers with virtually instant access to public opinions. "Bullet" approaches by well-organized but quantitatively minor factions ensure their "day in court." As George Will has pointed out,[1] the risk is that " . . . Congress becomes a marionette of opinion, a role devoid of dignity." These realities create an enormous challenge and opportunity for publicly supported science, which is much of science.

The major point of the articles in this chapter is that diverse publics must be involved if science is to thrive. Moreover, the tense interface between politics and science, described by Hanna, must be converted to productive collaboration. It is hard to communicate the various sciences to scientifically uninformed publics. Silverstone emphasizes that the reconstruction of science by recipients of information is extraordinarily complex and limiting. Indeed, effective communication of complex material is a growing science in itself.

It is support of fundamental science that is most fragile; pressures for application now dominate the agendas of major support agencies. Translating fundamental science into social value is particularly hard; how do we elicit support for an eclectic, unpredictable, painstakingly slow enterprise fraught with serendipity, ethical dilemmas, and occasional missteps. Moreover, direct public exposure has been anathema to many scientists, as it is time consuming, expensive, and diversionary. Furthermore, scientists tend to be data oriented, critical, and, as Jasanoff suggests, invested in unpredictability. There is, in fact, no one science and no stereotyped scientist; scientists often disagree among themselves, and public disagreements confuse. Yet there is merit in Ziman's position that these conflicts can yield good results—revealing the fundamental humanism of scientists and bringing science into the broader social context envisaged by Wynne and others.

Koshland put it well in a recent editorial,[2] "the key to good science policy is informed assent, in which legislators accept the need for scientific advice on the mechanism of achieving their goal, and scientists recognize that legislators have the right to set the strategic goals based on societal needs." The pursuit of fundamental science, one of our greatest cultural attributes, is inextricably linked to the public; it is precisely because of its enormous social promise that it must be supported, and that it can and should be presented for its ultimate social value.

There is cause for optimism: Research! America's recent surveys of registered voters in the state of Maryland reveal that most believe that more money should be spent on research aimed at preventing and treating disease. Fifty-six percent of those surveyed said that biomedical research was not getting enough support. Moreover, another survey conducted after a statewide public education program indicated a substantial increase in public support. These results are heartening for the future support of science and emphasize the importance of understanding through education.

When all is said and done, our publics need to know what we are doing, why we are doing it, and how we go about it. They must understand the benefits, risks, and costs of science.

Academic health centers are well positioned to lead the process, by deed and example. As major local, regional, and national resources, academic health centers are at the right intersection to educate and inform the public about science. We are "laboratories" of science and its critical application to the bedside (quality of life) and we have talented educators and communicators. But we cannot do it alone; we should support and collaborate with representative agencies.

We should (a) commit to effective public interaction, communication and education and learn to do them better, (b) involve the public in planning and decision-making where appropriate, and in addressing the many social and ethical issues we face and, (c) attend to research integrity and conflict of interest and avoid denials of fact.

There is a risk in this; public "desensitization" or, worse, negative reactions are possible outcomes. If we do it well, we will have much to gain.

References

1. Will GF. Rhetorical presidency. *Newsweek*. February 8, 1993: 74.
2. Koshland DE Jr. Basic Research (1). *Science*. 1993;259:291.

CHAPTER IX

Human Subjects: Protection, Policies, and Practice

ABSTRACTS AND EXCERPTS

■ Annas GJ. Changing the consent rules for Desert Storm. *N Engl J Med.* 1992;326:770-773.

Abstracted from information appearing in *NEJM*. Reprinted with permission of *The New England Journal of Medicine*.

Shortly before the beginning of Operation Desert Storm, during Desert Shield, the U.S. military sought a waiver of requirements for informed consent for the use of investigational drugs and vaccines on our troops in the Persian Gulf. . . . The legal maneuvering to revise consent regulations for wartime conditions provides a case study that highlights three separable issues: how easily the line between therapy and experimentation can become blurred; the differences between law and ethics; and the ethical obligations of physicians when the interests of their patients conflict with the interests of their employer.

In the fall of 1990, after the invasion of Kuwait by Iraq, the Department of Defense sought a waiver of the consent requirements in the Food and Drug

Administration's existing regulations governing human experimentation so that the military could administer investigational drugs and vaccines to the Desert Shield soldiers without their informed consent. The justification for the request was military expediency. In the words of the Department of Defense request: "In all peace time applications, we believe strongly in informed consent and its ethical foundations . . . but military combat is different." The department argued that informed consent under combat conditions was "not feasible" because some troops might refuse to consent, and the military could not tolerate such refusals because of "military combat exigencies." The FDA granted the request and issued a new general regulation, rule 23(d), that permits waivers on a drug-by-drug basis on the grounds that consent is "not feasible in a specific military operation involving combat or the immediate threat of combat."

What should physicians in the military do when asked to administer investigational agents without the informed consent of the soldiers? Even if such administration is legal (as the courts have ruled), many would find it unethical, and as the Nuremberg trials affirmed, "following orders" is no excuse for unethical conduct, even in combat.

The experience with rule 23(d) during Operation Desert Storm illustrates the difficulty of making distinctions between experimental inverventions and treatment, the difference between law (especially as enunciated by the courts during wartime) and ethics, and the potential conflicts between the best interests of a physician's patients and the interests of a physician's employer. Although it was designed to resolve these conflicts, rule 23(d) primarily served to highlight them and to reverse a 44-year policy of following the Nuremberg Code. The rule not only turned out to be militarily unncessary but also called into question the seriousness of the United States' human-rights agenda.

■ Brett A, Grodin M. Ethical aspects of human experimentation in health services research. *JAMA*. 1991;265:1854-1857.

Over the past several decades, ethical issues in human experimentation have received increasing attention in the medical literature. Most of this literature presumes a fairly standard conception of modern medical research, ie, the application of a therapeutic intervention to a group of persons with a specific diagnosis.

In contrast, the organizational, procedural, and economic aspects of health care provision have themselves become the focus of an enlarging body of research, termed *health services research*. Until recently, these studies were characterized primarily by either retrospective data collection or concurrent observation without experimental intervention. However, in an attempt to achieve greater scientific rigor, health services research has increasingly included prospective interventions involving human subjects.

The scope of this research is broad. At one end of the spectrum is research comparing alternative processes of rendering care for circumscribed clinical problems. . . . At the other end of the spectrum are large-scale randomized studies comparing complete systems of health care provision or financing, such as the RAND Health Insurance Experiment. Such studies have much in common with social experimentation in general. Between these two extremes are studies examining modifications of various components of health care provision (e.g., educational interventions to change physician behavior).

Despite the recent proliferation of such studies, health services research involving human subjects has not yet received the detailed bioethical scrutiny accorded to conventional research. We believe, however, that many health services studies present ethical problems warranting analysis as a special case within the broader context of human experimentation. This article explores those problems initially by using accepted ethical principles to highlight areas of contrast between conventional and health services research. We then analyze in greater detail three frequently problematic issues—defining research, cost containment, and informed consent. Finally, we will draw general conclusions about the ethical conduct of this research.

■ **Capron AM. Protection of research subjects: do special rules apply in epidemiology?** *Law, Medicine, and Health Care.* **1991;44:184-190.**

Reprinted with permission of the American Society of Law, Medicine & Ethics

Epidemiologists sometimes think of "ethics" as the source of those obstacles, which are believed to be embodied in the federal rules for the protection of research subjects—colloquially called 45 CFR Part 46—especially as they are interpreted by some institutional review boards (IRBs). . . . a major cause for confusion—despite provisions in the federal regulations intended to avoid (or at the very least, to speed up) inappropriate or unnecessary reviews—is that most IRBs, being used to reviewing clinical research, may impose expectations that are poorly suited to epidemiological research.

Yet before we dismiss ethics as nothing more than a cause of confusion and needless worry, I think we need to take a careful look at epidemiologists' ethical obligations to research subjects. In doing so, we should pay particular attention to three points: first, the difference between harming someone and wronging them; second, the role of informed consent in protecting against such wrongs; and third, the steps that can be taken to avoid or minimize particular harms associated with breaches of privacy and confidentiality.

At the heart of the protection of research subjects—through the federal regulations and the institutional review process—is concern for the physical well-being of the human beings who become involved in research projects.

Epidemiologic research can also involve the risk of harm, but it is typically of a different sort. . . . First, if data dealing with sensitive matters—either raw data or final results—can be linked to subjects, they may suffer social harm, such as ostracism or loss of employment. Second, even when individuals cannot be linked to information that is embarrassing (or worse), findings that paint an adverse picture of an entire population may eventuate in harm to that group, either directly or as a result of the adoption of laws or policies that have a negative impact on the welfare of group members.

How, then, have the law and ethics dealt with the risks of subjects being harmed? Primarily through two requirements: first, research must undergo review by a properly constituted body—usually called an IRB—which is supposed to foreclose studies that entail an unfavorable benefit-risk ratio, that are unfair in the distribution of risk in the population, or that do not provide for an adequate consent process.

The second means of protecting against harm is through requiring that investigators obtain the informed and voluntary consent of subjects before studying them.

. . . look at the functions that informed consent serves in research. Four stand out: promoting autonomy and self-determination, improving research, regularizing relationships between investigators and subjects, and protecting privacy. If these purposes can be met without individual subjects giving informed consent, then the omission of consent may be more ethically acceptable.

One alternative to individual consent might be to convene what Diane Baumrind has termed "peer consultants," selected from the study population. This would symbolize the investigator's respect for the human beings involved in the study as rational agents worthy of consideration; the peers would take the place of the subjects as collaborators in the design of the research, thereby approximating "self-determination"; and the information given to peers could serve the same function as informed consent in educating and reassuring the public.

A related—but distinct—strategy is to obtain permission for the use of records from their custodians.

Another alternative to prospective informed consent is to employ after-the-fact debriefing and informed veto. This gives subjects an opportunity to exercise self-determination as to at least part of the study, it symbolizes the researchers' respect for subjects' autonomy, and it removes the implication of coercion that inheres in nonvoluntary participation in research.

Finally, provisions could be made to compensate subjects for any injury they suffer as a result of being studied without their advance consent.

■ **Christakis NA, Panner MJ. Existing international ethical guidelines for human subjects research: some open questions. *Law, Medicine, and Health Care.* 1991;19:214-220.**

Reprinted with permission of the American Society of Law, Medicine & Ethics

International guidelines regarding ethics, and in particular the ethics of clinical research, are problematic on two broad levels. First, by asserting their universality, "international" guidelines obscure real and legitimate cross-cultural differences in ethical expectations. International guidelines seek to make homogeneous something which is not necessarily so. Second, existing guidelines are ambiguous about their objectives and purposes. On the one hand, guidelines are structured as a set of goals, largely aspirational in language and content. But on the other hand, such guidelines also suggest a normative function, providing a set of standards by which to judge and, if appropriate, sanction investigators' conduct.

. . . we will suggest an alternative approach to the development of guidelines, one that may facilitate the resolution of existing dilemmas.

. . . the conduct of trans-cultural clinical research, particularly in the context of the AIDS pandemic, has brought to light the theoretical limits of ethical guidelines—both in structure and in application. . . . It has become apparent that what existing standards of ethics are not is a mechanism for the resolution of conflicting ethical expectations under circumstances where the universality of the principles articulated within them is not recognized, or under circumstances where the principles articulated within the standards conflict with each other.

To address such situations, we propose a different type of international ethical guidelines, a type with a different objective. Such international guidelines, instead of emphasizing the c*ontent* of research ethics, would emphasize the *process* in which any disagreement over content might be settled. Such "procedural" guidelines would help to settle, through negotiation, possible conflicts between disparate ethical ideals.

We would recommend a two-step process through which 1) international guidelines are subject to ratification within each nation and 2) a new type of international ethical code is developed which outlines dispute resolution principles for conflicting ethical expectations.

Not only do we believe that this will facilitate socially useful research in a fair way, but we believe that ultimately it will lead to a more expansive and just vision of human subjects research.

■ DeGregorio MW. Is tamoxifen chemoprevention worth the risk in healthy women? *The Journal of NIH Research.* 1992;4:84-87.

Reprinted with permission from *The Journal of NIH Research.*

The National Surgical Adjuvant Breast and Bowel Project Group (NSABP) has initiated a clinical trial sponsored by the National Cancer Institute to determine the value of tamoxifen for preventing breast cancer in 16,000 healthy women deemed to be at high risk of developing breast cancer. Tamoxifen is a nonsteroidal antiestrogen that competitively blocks estrogen receptors in breast cancer cells, thus producing an antiproliferative effect. In primary breast cancer, following surgery, adjuvant tamoxifen therapy produces a 20-percent reduction in disease recurrence at 10 years. Tamoxifen has also been shown to produce clinical benefits in at least 33 percent of women with metastatic breast cancer—independent of hormone-receptor status—and 50 percent of women with estrogen-receptor positive breast tumors. Tamoxifen has been touted as a relatively safe drug with an acceptable toxicity profile when used to treat patients with breast cancer, even though a small percentage of women develop major toxicities—including thromboembolitic events and secondary endometrial tumors. Tamoxifen therapy is associated with several other manageable toxicities, such as hot flashes, menstrual irregularities, and vaginal discharge. Virtually all patients with metastatic disease develop tamoxifen resistance, which is manifested in clinical tumor progression. Although tamoxifen is associated with adverse side effects and a risk of developing resistant breast cancer during the course of therapy, its clinical benefits outweigh the risks in patients with metastatic breast cancer or a history of breast cancer. However, the proposed benefit of tamoxifen as a chemopreventive agent in healthy women is likely to be significantly reduced after both the risk of side effects and the development of tamoxifen-resistant breast tumors are taken into account.

■ Dickens B. Issues in preparing ethical guidelines for epidemiological studies. *Law, Medicine and Health Care.* 1991;19:175-183.

Reprinted with permission of the American Society of Law, Medicine & Ethics

A movement has occurred in the field of public or population health . . . to develop guidelines for the ethical review of epidemiological studies, including public health and preventive health care initiatives. This is fuelled both by an emerging trend towards professionalism among many epidemiologists, and by sensitivities about prevalence studies of AIDS and HIV infection in particular populations.

Accordingly, in 1989 CIOMS [Council for International Organizations of Medical Sciences] undertook to prepare guidelines for the ethical review of epidemiological studies, which have been proposed in the fall of 1991 for longer-term consideration by those they are intended to serve. . . . CIOMS has long had special interests in health care in developing countries and was concerned to ensure that perspectives of both developed and developing countries would shape the guidelines. In the course of this exercise, a number of difficult issues became apparent that challenge the understanding of research ethics developed in clinical research, and that are distinctive to population health studies.

An initial issue was whether the guidelines were to be designed to govern the practice of epidemiology, or epidemiologists.

A further initial issue was whether the guidelines should, like the Nuremberg, Helsinki and related codes, limit themselves to health research, or extend to practice or surveillance programs, and whether indeed the distinction exists in epidemiology.

[Other issues include: consent and approval, confidentiality, justice, harms and wrongs, preventing injury, avoidance of conflicts of interest, and respect for culture.]

■ **Dresser R. Wanted: single, white male for medical research.**
Hastings Center Report. **1992;22:24-29.**

In June 1990, congressional investigators issued a startling report. The General Accounting Office revealed that despite a 1986 federal policy to the contrary, women continued to be seriously underrepresented in biomedical research study populations. According to the National Institutes of Health, this practice "has resulted in significant gaps in [our] knowledge" of diseases that affect both men and women. In short, many of the important human health data generated by the modern biomedical research revolution are data about men.

Moreover, the customary research subject not only is male, but is a white male. African-Americans, Latinos, and other racial and ethnic groups have typically been excluded from studies, again in spite of a formal NIH guideline encouraging the inclusion of such groups in study populations.

As a result of the past overrepresentation of white men in research populations, physicians now frequently lack adequate evidence on whether women and people of color will be helped, harmed, or not affected at all by numerous therapies now endorsed as promoting "human health."

The current disparity between the health information we have about white males and the information we have about women and people of color contravenes basic ethical principles governing human experimentation. Most clearly violated is the principle of beneficence, which holds that biomedical research should be designed to maximize benefit and minimize harm. . . . When diseases disproportionately affecting women and people of color are given low funding priority, knowledge that could alter current ineffective or detrimental routine medical care is never produced.

The harm produced by the exclusionary practices is not easily dismissed. Simple extrapolation from white males to everyone else can be dangerous.

Scientists and policymakers must recognize that the choice is not whether to protect women and people of color from research risks. Instead, the choice is whether to expose some consenting members of these groups to risk in the closely monitored research setting, or to expose many more of them to risk in the clinical setting without these safeguards, which is the result of the current approach.

NIH officials and biomedical researchers have, consciously or unconsciously, defined the white male as the normal, representative human being. From this perspective, the goal of advancing human health can be achieved by studying the white male human model.

Perhaps there was also a more insidious influence on the decisions about study populations. At least some scientists and government officials might have believed it was not important even to find out whether data from studies on white males applied to women and people of color. We cannot dismiss the possibility that the exclusionary practice reflected implicit social worth judgments on who ought to have priority in obtaining the fruits of biomedical research.

The immediate task for scientists and government officials involves revamping study design and reordering funding priorities to remedy past exclusionary practices.

Second is the challenge to use the emerging knowledge about biological differences for the benefit of historically disadvantaged groups.

■ **Gostin L. Ethical principles for the conduct of human subject research: population-based research and ethics.** *Law, Medicine, and Health Care.* **1991;19:191-201.**

Reprinted with permission of the American Society of Law, Medicine & Ethics

[Three] ethical principles [respect for persons, beneficence, and justice] have found expression in international guidelines for the conduct of clinical research, and have been codified in national statutes and regulations, particularly in the developed world.

Ethical principles help support autonomy and self-determination, protect the vulnerable, and promote the welfare and equality of human beings. But traditional ethics focuses primarily on individual rights and duties, and does not always see individuals as part of wider social orders and communities. A person dominated medical ethic is insufficient for the task of setting moral and human rights boundaries around the conduct of research on populations.

This paper provides a halting first step in organizing a set of ethical guidelines for the conduct of population-based research, surveillance and practice. These principles are not distinct from, but an expansion of, traditional ethics.

Population based research, surveillance, and practice can have extraordinary benefits and risks. The potential for human good, measured in improvement of health and decreased morbidity and mortality from population-based research and practice represents one of the great triumphs of science in the 20th century. But, the potential to cause harm to human beings and the groups they comprise is also much greater.

Foundational principles must be developed to protect the dignity and integrity of all populations including vulnerable populations which are non-dominant, poor, disenfranchised, compromised, persecuted, or restricted. This paper enunciates five such principles: (i) the overriding imperative to protect the health and well-being of populations, (ii) respect for populations and their right to self-determination, (iii) protection of vulnerable populations and the need for special justifications for research, (iv) protecting the privacy, integrity, and self-esteem of populations, and (v) the equitable distribution of benefits to populations and the importance of building infra-structure.

■ Hellman S, Hellman DS. Of mice but not men: problems of the randomized clinical trial. *N Engl J Med.* 1991;324:1585-1589.

Abstracted from information appearing in *NEJM*. Reprinted with permission of the *New England Journal of Medicine*.

As medicine has become increasingly scientific and less accepting of unsupported opinion or proof by anecdote, the randomized controlled clinical trial has become the standard technique for changing diagnostic or therapeutic methods. The use of this technique creates an ethical dilemma. Researchers participating in such studies are required to modify their ethical commitments to individual patients and do serious damage to the concept of the physician as a practicing, empathetic professional who is primarily concerned with each patient as an individual.

The randomized clinical trial requires doctors to act simultaneously as physicians and as scientists. This puts them in a difficult and sometimes untenable ethical position. The conflicting moral demands arising from the use of the randomized clinical trial reflect the classic conflict between rights-based moral theories and utilitarian ones.

. . . the randomized clinical trial routinely asks physicians to sacrifice the interests of their particular patients for the sake of the study and that of the information that it will make available for the benefit of society. This practice is ethically problematic.

If the physician has no opinion about whether the new treatment is acceptable, then random assignment is ethically acceptable, but such lack of enthusiasm for the new treatment does not augur well for either the patient or the study. Alternatively, the treatment may show promise of beneficial results but also present a risk of undesirable complications. When the physician believes that the severity and likelihood of harm and good are evenly balanced, randomization may be ethically acceptable. If the physician has no preference for either treatment (is in a state of equipoise), then randomization is acceptable. If, however, he or she believes that the new treatment may be either more or less successful or more or less toxic, the use of randomization is not consistent with fidelity to the patient.

Even if randomized clinical trials were much better than any alternative, however, the ethical dilemmas they present may put their use at variance with the primary obligations of the physician. . . . Techniques appropriate to the laboratory may not be applicable to humans. We must develop and use alternative methods for acquiring clinical knowledge.

■ Ijsselmuiden CB, Faden RR. Research and informed consent in Africa—another look. *N Engl J Med.* 1992;326:830-834.

Abstracted from information appearing in *NEJM*. Reprinted with permission of the *New England Journal of Medicine*.

The current practice of requiring the informed consent of research subjects is relatively new.

Although both the Nuremberg Code of 1948 and the Declaration of Helsinki of 1964 made the consent of subjects a central requirement of ethical research, it was not until the mid-1970s that the practice of requiring informed consent for medical research became conventional in the West. . . . The fundamental justification for requiring consent from human subjects as a matter of U.S. public policy is best stated in the Belmont Report of 1978, which bases the obligation to obtain consent on the ethical principle of respect for persons.

This strong emphasis on respect for autonomy is, however, neither unchallenged in the United States itself nor necessarily accepted elsewhere in the world, including Western Europe and Africa. The challenge centers on the validity of applying ethical guidelines for research that are accepted in one part of the world to a different cultural setting.

The most fundamental argument against modifying the obligation of researchers to obtain informed consent from individual subjects is that such an obligation expresses important and basic moral values that are universally applicable, regardless of variations in cultural practice.

Proposals to modify informed-consent requirements must take account of the complex motivation behind decisions to conduct research in the developing world rather than in the West.

Although careful reflection by Western scientists about the ethics of conducting research in Africa is essential, it is no substitute for the establishment of standards and practices by Africans themselves. . . . The years of public debate and governmental consultation that led to the Belmont Report in the United States are an example waiting to be emulated elsewhere.

■ Osborne NG, Feit MD. The use of race in medical research. *JAMA*. 1992;267:275-279.

When race is used as a variable in research, there is a tendency to assume that the results obtained are a manifestation of the biology of racial differences; race as a variable implies that a genetic reason may explain differences in incidence, severity, or outcome of medical conditions. Researchers, without saying so, lead readers to assume that certain racial groups have a special predisposition, risk, or susceptibility to the illnesses studied. Since this presupposition is seldom warranted, this kind of comparison may be taken to represent a subtle form of racism. But in any case, although there are ethical problems with the search for genetic reasons to explain certain types of diseases, the scientific pitfalls that stand in the way of ethnic research are formidable since racial status is highly correlated with social, economic, and political factors. We will explore the practical problems and examine the consequences of using race as a category in medical research.

The concept of race is, at best, elusive. There is no accepted scientific definition of race. Racial definitions (and connotations) depend on location, social class, and nationality. Race is not a dichotomous variable such as gender or marital status. . . . To establish scientific credibility, authors must solve several difficult practical problems. How white is white? At what point in one's ancestry does race change?

Is a person who has only one grandparent of another race defined or categorized the same as one who has one great-grandparent or two great-grandparents? What happens if two grandparents are white, one is black, and another Asian? To make matters worse, the concept of race varies with geography. Defining someone as black in Louisiana may be quite different from definitions in Wisconsin, Latin America, or South Africa.

The category of race in research is likely to be complicated by a problem of perception. The issue is not merely academic. Medical attitudes and ideas have social, economic, and therapeutic consequences. The social consequences of racial comparisons in medical publications may depend more on the perceptions that adverse comparisons reinforce in society than on the accuracy of the data, the intent of the authors, or the correctness of their interpretation.

When scientists identify race as a marker for social deprivation, cultural attitudes, or any other determinants of disease, they should be required to follow their preliminary reports with more detailed analyses as a condition for publication. A detailed analysis of the hypotheses used to justify race as a category for research may then lead to a meaningful recognition of social, economic, political, and cultural factors that contribute to the risk of disease.

■ **Passamani E. Clinical trials—are they ethical?** *N Engl J Med.* **1991;324:1589-1592.**

Abstracted from information appearing in *NEJM*. Reprinted with permission of the *New England Journal of Medicine*.

Clinical trials have . . . become a preferred means of evaluating an ever increasing flow of innovative diagnostic and therapeutic maneuvers. The randomized, double-blind clinical trial is a powerful technique because of the efficiency and credibility associated with treatment comparisons involving randomized concurrent controls.

. . . randomized trials are in fact the most scientifically sound and ethically correct means of evaluating new therapies. There is potential conflict between the roles of physician and physician-scientist, and for this reason society has created mechanisms to ensure that the interests of individual patients are served should they elect to participate in a clinical trial.

To summarize, randomized clinical trials are an important element in the spectrum of biomedical research. Not all questions can or should be addressed by this technique; feasibility, cost, and the relative importance of the issues to be addressed are weighed by investigators before they elect to proceed. Properly carried out, with informed consent, clinical equipoise, and a design adequate to answer the question posed, randomized clinical trials protect physicians and their patients from therapies that are ineffective or toxic. Physicians and their patients must be clear about the vast gulf separating promising and proved therapies. The only reliable way to make this distinction in the face of incomplete information about pathophysiology and treatment mechanism is to experiment, and this will increasingly involve randomized trials. The alternative—a retreat to older methods—is unacceptable.

■ Twenty years after: the legacy of the Tuskegee syphilis study. *Hastings Center Report.* 1992;22:29-32.

This year marks the twentieth anniversary of the end of the Tuskegee syphilis study, one of the more notorious episodes in the history of human subjects research in the United States. Begun in 1932, the study was purportedly designed to determine the natural history of untreated syphilis in a population of some 400 black men in Tuskegee, Alabama. The research subjects, all of whom had syphilis at the time they were enrolled in the study, were matched against 200 uninfected controls.

Though the subjects had received the standard heavy metals therapy available in 1932, they were denied antibiotic therapy when it became clear in the 1940s that penicillin was a safe and effective treatment for the disease. Subjects were recruited with misleading promises of "special free treatment" (actually spinal taps done without anesthesia to study the neurological effects of syphilis), and were enrolled without their informed consent. Disclosure of the ongoing research in the popular media in 1972 led to the termination of the study and ultimately to the National Research Act of 1974, which mandates institutional review board (IRB) approval of all federally funded proposed research with human subjects.

As final payments are being made under the agreement that settled a class action lawsuit brought on behalf of the subjects of the Tuskegee study, the articles that follow look at different facets of Tuskegee's legacy. Should the results of an immorally conducted study continue to serve as the "gold standard" in our clinical understanding of syphilis? How shall we strike a balance between protecting vulnerable classes of subjects already discriminated against and seeing that minorities are adequately represented in—and reap the benefits of—clinical trials? What lingering meanings does Tuskegee have in the African American community, and how do those meanings affect current efforts not only to conduct biomedical research, but also to provide effective health care in the community? And finally, what messages do race, or other kinds of difference, carry in our culture?

■ Caplan AL. When evil intrudes. *Hastings Center Report*. 1992;22:29-32.

Syphilis continues to challenge America's and the world's medical, public health, and moral resources.

. . . the continuing invocation of the findings of the Tuskegee study by those who diagnose, study, or treat syphilis shows that it is sometimes impossible to avoid a confrontation with the questions of the ethics of relying on knowledge obtained in the course of immoral research.

. . . the Tuskegee study was and remains a key source of information about the diagnosis, signs, symptoms, and course of syphilis.

The acceptance of the Tuskegee study findings as valid refutes the argument that bad ethics is always incompatible with valid science . . . . But even if it were wrong to cite data acquired by immoral means there is simply no way to purge the knowledge gained in the Tuskegee study from biomedicine.

Given that the study played a crucial role in causing Americans to rethink the ethics of human experimentation, it would seem morally incumbent upon those who discuss its findings in the context of textbooks and review articles to allot some space for a discussion of the ethical problems associated with it.

If no place is made for discussions of the morality of studies such as Tuskegee, the research community may become complacent about the importance of its responsibilities toward human subjects at the same time as the public comes to believe that good science cannot emerge from immoral research.

■ Edgar H. Outside the community. *Hastings Center Report*. 1992;22:32-35.

. . . I should like to describe some aspects of the legal landscape of the Tuskegee litigation. The injustices done to the participants did not fit easily into the framework of an adjudicable lawsuit. . . . Did the act permit recovery for harm done between 1932 to 1945 to people (many of whom were dead by 1946), on the theory that there had been an ongoing project whose success depended upon keeping the facts secret from the participants? Second, could unwitting (and unwilling) service in an experiment give rise to a contract claim against the government, or even a claim that government had taken property and owed compensation? Third, what relevancy, if any, did Nuremberg have?

The Tuskegee study was . . . a major force in the development of American bioethics. Among other things, it was a direct cause of the National Research Act in 1974, which required the establishment of institutional review boards at institutions receiving federal grants.

Apart from its violation of human rights, the Tuskegee study was a serious incident of what is now called "science misconduct.". . . not only . . . [was] the study . . . ethically wrong measured by the ethical standards of the 1970s, but . . . it had been, from the start, a program built upon deception.

The central fact about the forty-year study was that its scientific rationale made no sense.

One irony about Tuskegee is that the study was racist to the core, in that no such program could possibly have continued so long but for the central fact that participants were African Americans.

On the issue of racial impact of the disease, the physicians involved unquestionably believed both before the study and as a result of the study's data that syphilis does affect different groups differently.

There has been a sea-change in attitude about such matters today. At present, any assertion of group difference is always a potentially explosive issue. . . . Yet what the Tuskegee doctors could contemplate—group differences—will be forced upon the medical world in the effort to understand problems ranging from why some people get lung cancer while others do not, to how come the French eat so much fat and do not get our rates of heart disease. Indeed, the fact that groups may be different . . . may have major implications for how we appraise "research" as opposed to "experimental therapies," for we draw lines between these categories more sharply than the reality makes desirable.

To acknowledge those differences, while insisting on their irrelevance to respect for individual dignity and equality of right, is a challenge we shall have to face.

■ King PA. The dangers of difference. *Hastings Center Report.* 1992;22:35-38.

The social and ethical issues that the experiment poses for medicine, particularly for medicine's relationship with African Americans, are still not broadly understood, appreciated, or even remembered. Yet a significant aspect of the Tuskegee experiment's legacy is that in a racist society that incorporates beliefs about the inherent inferiority of African Americans in contrast with the superior status of whites, any attention to the question of differences that may exist is likely to be pursued in a manner that burdens rather than benefits African Americans.

The racism that played a central role in this tragedy continues to infect even our current well-intentioned efforts to reverse the decline in health status of African Americans.

The argument that provided critical support for the experiment was that the natural course of untreated syphilis in blacks and whites was not the same.

Recognizing and taking account of racial differences that have historically been utilized to burden and exploit African Americans poses a dilemma. . . . Because medicine is pragmatic, it will recognize racial differences if dong so will promote health goals. As a consequence, potential harms that might result from attention to racial differences tend to be overlooked, minimized, or viewed as problems beyond the purview of medicine.

The question of whether (and how) to take account of racial differences has recently been raised in the context of the current AIDS epidemic.

Understanding how, or indeed whether, race correlates with disease is a very complicated problem. Race itself is a confusing concept with both biological and social connotations.

In the wake of Tuskegee and, in more recent times, the stigma and discrimination that resulted from screening for sickle cell trait (a genetic condition that occurs with greater frequency among African Americans), researchers have been reluctant to explore associations between race and disease. There is increasing recognition, however, of evidence of heightened resistance or vulnerability to disease along racial lines.

Clearly, priority should be given to exploring the possible social, cultural, and environmental determinants of disease before targeting the study of hypotheses that involve biological differences between blacks and whites.

■ **Jones JH. The Tuskegee legacy: AIDS and the black community.**
Hastings Center Report. 1992;22:38-40.

No scientific experiment inflicted more damage on the collective psyche of black Americans than the Tuskegee study. . . . Confronted with the experiment's moral bankruptcy, many blacks lost faith in the government and no longer believed health officials who spoke on matters of public concern. Consequently, when a terrifying new plague swept the land in the 1980s and 1990s, the Tuskegee study predisposed many blacks to distrust health authorities, a fact many whites had difficulty understanding.

For many blacks, the Tuskegee study became a symbol of their mistreatment by the medical establishment, a metaphor for deceit, conspiracy, malpractice, and neglect, if not outright racial genocide.

Health officials who worked in black communities reported that the Tuskegee study had spawned a legacy of suspicion and distrust toward public health authorities.

Not surprisingly, then, many health officials encountered difficulties when they tried to study AIDS in black communities.

As a symbol of racism and medical malfeasance, the Tuskegee study may never move the nation to action, but it can change the way Americans view illness. Hidden within the anger and anguish of those who decry the experiment is a plea for government authorities and medical officials to hear the fears of people whose faith has been damaged, to deal with their concerns directly, and to acknowledge the link between public health and community trust.

COMMENTARY

Carol A. Aschenbrener

T he basic ethical principles of beneficence, nonmalefi-
cence, autonomy, and justice are rooted in antiquity.
The refinements of informed consent and protection
of human subjects, however, are post-World War II
developments. Atrocities of medical research on prisoners of war prompted reflection on the need to protect human
subjects, and the rising standard of living in the West gave society
the time to more deeply consider what "respect for persons" demands.

The Nuremberg Code stressed voluntary consent of the human
subjects as "absolutely essential." (Rule 1). This voluntary consent
entailed informing by the treating or investigating physician and
consenting by the patient or subject. The ramifications and the
analytical dissection of this requirement of informed consent have
dominated the medical ethics literature for more than 30 years.
Initially, much of the debate centered on the recognition that individuals with diminished autonomy, such as prisoners, children, and
the incompetent, required special protection. Using the duty to "do
no harm" as basis, discussions of informed consent emphasized
identification of groups and individuals that should be excluded as
research subjects because they could not comprehend the risks and
benefits or were vulnerable to coercion that restricted voluntary
consent.

The rise of individualism, associated with the civil rights and
feminist movements of the 1960s, was accompanied by an increased
emphasis on autonomy. Informed consent was linked to the right
to self-determination and the focus shifted to full disclosure of risks
and benefits. In February 1966, the U.S. Surgeon General issued
the first policy statement requiring independent review of measures
for protection of human subjects, including informed consent and
assessment of risks and potential benefits, prior to conducting re-

search supported by the United States Public Health Service. Subsequent regulations of the Department of Health, Education, and Welfare established Institutional Review Boards (1973) and elaborated ethical and legal duties of investigators.

In the 1970s, issues of justice commanded increasing attention. Physicians struggled with criteria for allocation of scarce resources such as renal dialysis machines and organs for transplantation. In 1978, the National Commission for the Protection of Human Subjects of Biomedical and Behavioral Research issued a report calling for just treatment of research subjects.[1] That report cautioned against taking advantage of vulnerable groups and emphasized the necessity to exclude as subjects those members of groups that were unlikely to benefit from the results.

Public awareness of the impact of race, ethnicity, socioeconomic and educational status on informed consent has been slow to develop. As centers of scientific and ethical inquiry, academic health centers have a responsibility to address the protection of individuals with particular vulnerability. This includes members of vulnerable populations, that is, "individuals or groups who are non-dominant, subservient or subject to restrictions in the culture where they live."

In his excellent treatise Ethics and Regulations of Clinical Research, Levine emphasizes the element of negotiation in informed consent.[2] Katz illustrates this interchange of informed consent with a dance metaphor that entails invitation by the investigator, dialogue between investigator and invited subject, and eventual acceptance or declination of invitation by the subject. It is essential that the nature of the invitation and the dialogue be shaped according to the context of the research and the special characteristics of invited subjects. The investigator seeking consent must have sufficient understanding of the culture and ethnicity of subjects to identify and remove barriers to voluntary consent. Are there cultural taboos that might be violated in the research protocol? Do members of vulnerable groups feel free to question the invitation or express discomfort and pain? Great care must be taken with those people who have limited fluency in English.

With increasing emphasis on health promotion and disease prevention, there is demand for population-based research to establish epidemiologic patterns, to evaluate behavioral modification strategies, and to measure health outcomes. Such research has the potential for improving care for underserved populations. However, the results of such research, when strategied by race, culture, or gender could also be used to reinforce existing bias. Studies that report rates of HIV infection by race stigmatize those particular groups. In addition, through their failure to focus on other vulnerable groups, including women and children, such studies may compromise treatment for these people. Great care must be taken to search for root causes. For example, the 1988 National Household Survey of Drug Abuse concluded that crack cocaine smoking is more prevalent among African Americans and Hispanic Americans than among Caucasians. The results of a recent study, which restratified respondents according to neighborhood risk sets, strongly suggest that the differences are not race-based but related to environmental factors such as social condition and availability of crack cocaine.[3]

The recent requirements of the National Institutes of Health (NIH) for the inclusion of women and members of minority groups in clinical research emphasize the duty of researchers to include groups that either might benefit or that might be harmed if research results are applied without understanding of gender and racial differences. It is less clear what duty investigators have to search for existing bias in treatment. A recent study of coronary artery angioplasty and CABG demonstrates that both procedures have higher mortality for women and both are performed 2-3 times more frequently on men. Since their introduction, these very costly procedures have been performed far more frequently on white men. Will clinicians seek explanations for the differential mortality in the experience of surgeons and in modifiable sex-based differences of patients or will they assume that the procedure is too risky for women and avoid recommending it?

Levine notes that one purpose of informing subjects about the purpose of research is to give them the opportunity to decline invitation if they do not share or value the goals of that research. This is particularly relevant with regard to outcomes research that is directed at cost containment. Historically, the goal of clinical research has been to alleviate suffering, if not for the subject at least for future beneficiaries. With some health services research, the suffering targeted for alleviation is economic, not physical or psychological. The beneficiary is society, not the individual.

Most major proposals for health care reform place great emphasis on outcomes research as a means of controlling costs. How will the interests of patients be protected when cost control is the goal? Patients are known to be more likely to accept randomization to a clinical trial if their physician asserts that there is no treatment considered more effective. Under capitated systems, how will physicians avoid conflict of interest in evaluating treatments that might be more expensive to provide? With federally funded outcomes research, will investigators have potential conflicts of interest similar to that which many assert occurs when drug trials are funded by pharmaceutical companies? How will investigators balance the duty to protect their subjects with admonitions to control costs? Will investigators fear that their ability to compete for federal funding will be compromised by studies that establish expensive treatments as more effective?

The ongoing clinical trials of high-dose chemotherapy combined with autologous bone marrow transplant for treatment of metastatic breast cancer illustrate some ethical concerns that may be exacerbated in a capitated system. Some insurance companies cover this new therapy only if patients are enrolled in a clinical trial. Can consent be voluntary under such circumstances? Will insurers be forced to confront the peer review system in determining when treatment is conventional and subject to reimbursement? What will be the roles for insurers and peer review? Will more data be required for treatments that are more expensive than standard therapy? Will less expensive treatments be adopted without equally rigorous peer review? How will cost affect decisions to stop trials when efficacy is proven? Some insurers cover clinical trials only at institutions where insurers have existing contracts for negotiated rates. In a new system, particularly a capitated one, will the incentives be such that institutions will avoid testing new therapies that may be more expensive or may jeopardize their insurance contracts or their fiscal well-being?

Michael Friedman, M.D., associate director of cancer therapy evaluation at the National Cancer Institute was quoted as saying, "We have a profound responsibility to women with breast cancer today. But we have an equal responsibility to make sure the therapies we prescribe tomorrow are the most rational, effective, and affordable ones."[4] Confronted with the inescapable need to face the cost of idealistic social programs, society may need to rebalance individual good with the common good. It may be necessary to rebalance justice and autonomy, but this should be done explicitly through social policy rather than implicitly or unwittingly through cost-focused outcomes research. To assert that the investigator has an equal duty to promote the welfare of patients and to achieve cost control is to confuse the duties of physicians and scientists with the duties of government. It is essential that physicians and other clinical investigators remain focused on beneficence and autonomy and let citizens and policymakers grapple with justice.

References

1. The National Commission for the Protection of Human Subjects of Biomedical and Behavioral Research: The Belmont Report: Ethical Principles and Guidelines for the Protection of Human Subjects of Research. DHEW Publication No. (OS) 78-0012, Appendix I: Washington, DC; 1978.
2. Levine RJ. *Ethics and Regulation of Clinical Research.* New Haven, Conn: Yale University Press;1986.
3. Lillie-Blanton M, Anthony JC, Schuster CR. Probing the meaning of racial/ethnic group comparisons in crack cocaine smoking. *JAMA.* 1993;269:993-997.
4. Meyer H. Breast study woes preview reform barriers. *AMNews.* Mar. 9, 1993;1.

COMMENTARY

David Korn

T he articles and papers selected for this chapter are all concerned with the issue of experimental studies on human subjects, and they pose an extraordinary array of challenging questions that range from fundamental ethical principles and the interpretations of pertinent law to cherished doctrines of scientific methodology. Our existing ethical and legal framework for the protection of human subjects in research owes its modern origins to the profound outpouring of public revulsion in response to revelations of "medical experiments" that were carried out by German doctors on concentration camp inmates and other incarcerated unfortunates during World War II. The key documents that constitute this framework include the Nuremberg Code of 1947, the Declaration of Helsinki, originally promulgated in 1964 and subsequently modified, and the guidelines published in 1982 by the Council for International Organizations of Medical Sciences (CIOMS). These documents share in common a foundation on the three basic ethical principles of autonomy, beneficence, and justice, and they prominently articulate respect for the individual person, the dignity of each human life, and the overarching requirement of informed consent.

These papers raise provocative questions about these principles, their applicability and their application in a host of different circumstances that extend from the exigencies of wartime combat, to the differential treatment of experimental populations, whether subtle or explicit, advertent or inadvertent, based on race, socioeconomic stratum, gender, or nationality. One might anticipate that these issues would present themselves most commonly, at least for purposes of pedagogy, with respect to clinical studies that involve large populations in underdeveloped countries; in fact, they are prominently at play and readily discernible within the United States. Let me offer several contemporary examples to illustrate this point.

The Tuskegee study of the natural history of syphilis in black males stands as a permanent blot on our national escutcheon and a discomfiting reminder that one does not have to seek out Third World countries or totalitarian regimes to find egregious examples of abuses of human subjects in research. The revelation of the Tuskegee study in the early 1970s led to widely publicized congressional hearings to the formation by Congress of a blue ribbon commission that developed the foundation of ethical principles governing research on human subjects in this country, and to the passage of the National Research Act in 1974, which enacted in statute the requirement for institution-based, multidisciplinary ethics committees (which we now know as IRBs) to approve and oversee all research studies involving human subjects in the United States.

As several of the papers point out, the Tuskegee study has left this country with some very unfortunate legacies. Particularly within the African-American community, but doubtless within other non-white American populations as well, there persists a deep-seated distrust of our medical establishment, which remains, as we approach the mid-1990s, a predominantly white male enterprise and culture. One salient example of the contemporary consequences of this legacy has to do with organ transplantation. In spite of a recent plethora of well-publicized initiatives, waiting lists of eligible organ recipients have steadily increased, and the national supply of organ donors has been distressingly flat for several years now.

The growth in numbers of potential recipients, of course, results from remarkable advancements in the science and technology of organ transplantation in infants, children, and adults; but as this scientific and technological capability has progressively expanded, the number of organ donors has not responded, and the rate-limiting factor of organ supply has become a strangling choke collar in every major organ transplantation program in the United States.

Analysis of potential and actual donor populations by our national system of Organ Procurement Organizations (OPOs) has revealed marked discrepancies in donation rates among different racial and ethnic sub-populations. Specifically, the probability of consent is far lower among African American, Hispanic American and Asian American populations than it is among whites. Comparable problems have been well recognized in bone marrow transplantation, where substantial efforts are now underway to develop specific registries within the black and Latino populations.

Many conferences and published studies have documented these problems and evaluated their causes, and consistent among these is the prominent theme of distrust of the medical establishment. Interestingly, that distrust seems not to be directed at the white medical establishment exclusively. For example, at Howard University in Washington, D.C., a robust program of kidney transplantation involving predominantly African-American recipients is overwhelmingly dependent on white organ donors from the surrounding area. The legacy of Tuskegee indeed runs deep in the American consciousness.

In recent years, this country has witnessed a crescendo of concern over sundry issues relating to gender discrimination and gender inequity. Among these issues, one that is particularly pertinent to the theme of this chapter is the systematic failure to include reasonable numbers of women (or ethnic minorities, for that matter) in a host of federally funded clinical trials involving large populations, prolonged periods of study, and substantial costs. Prominent among these, but not exclusively limited to them, have been long-term studies concerned with the natural history, prevention, and treatment of major cardiovascular diseases. In response to this problem, statutory and regulatory remedies have been promulgated that now specifically require the inclusion of women (as well as of members of minority populations) in all federally sponsored clinical trials, unless their exclusion is explicitly mandated by the nature of the scientific problem under study.

The current focus on this basic issue of equity is welcome and long overdue. On the other hand, as is not uncommon in governmental responses to perceived injustices, there is always the danger of compensatory excesses. A few examples are informative. Our national system of affiliated medical centers of the U.S. Department of Veterans Affairs (VA) has made many important contributions to the fund of biomedical knowledge through its unique capacity to organize and conduct large-scale clinical trials. Patient populations in VA hospitals have until relatively recently been almost exclusively male. Accordingly, the clinical trials conducted in the VA medical system have predominantly involved male subjects. In a recent episode, a proposed study that originated in an affiliated VA medical center and had been extremely well evaluated by peer review ran into serious difficulties with respect to funding from the National Institutes of Health (NIH) because of the small fraction of women subjects who were incorporated into the study. By involving affiliated non-VA institutions in the study, the principal investigator had made a diligent effort to enlist women subjects, but the proportion remained low. Given the circumstances of this case, unwillingness to fund this proposal on the grounds of gender distribution would seem to represent an abuse of administrative authority that reflects more zeal than common sense.

Another example concerns a contentious and highly politicized clinical trial, in which a group of respected investigators proposed a long-term study to evaluate the effects of sharply reduced dietary fat content on the incidence of breast cancer in postmenopausal women. The study, which is now part of the expansive Women's Health initiative that has been launched by the NIH, was originally submitted to the National Cancer Institute. It was reviewed on three separate occasions by the National Cancer Advisory Board, which voted nearly unanimously on each occasion not to fund the study. The disputed issues in this large, expensive, and long-term investigation, were many and centered on serious questions of concept and methodology about which the scientific community was sharply divided.

One particular aspect of that case, however, involved an ethical issue that is pertinent to this discussion. A major concern of the board was the statistical power of the study to discern significant differences in outcomes between the experimental and control populations, even given generous assumptions of population size, duration of study, and financial costs. The study design required the experimental group to maintain an extremely low dietary fat intake for a period of many years and the control population to maintain the dietary fat intake now typical of the average American population, which was a level twice as high as that proposed in the experimental group.

The board was troubled by the increasing public attention being directed at the dangers of high fat intake and the heightened intensity of public exhortation for Americans to sharply reduce their dietary fat intake. Indeed, while the proposal was still under evaluation, the U.S. Department of Health and Human Services issued a new guideline urging that the dietary fat intake of Americans be reduced by 25 percent or the amount that, if achieved, would have halved the difference in fat intake anticipated between the experimental and control populations. Moreover, it was clear that if, in response to this public pressure, the average dietary fat intake were to decline over the many years proposed for the study—thereby narrowing the difference between experimental and control groups— the statistical power of the trial to discern significant differences in cancer incidence would have been progressively attenuated and become highly problematic.

A question was raised about the ethical obligation of the National Cancer Institute and the applicant investigators regarding informed consent for the tens of thousands of control women who were to be enrolled in the study and followed for periods of at least 8 to 10 years, and probably much longer. Did the investigators and the federal sponsor not have a positive duty to intervene with the control population and encourage these women to change their dietary behavior in accordance with the new federal guidelines? And how should one evaluate such a lengthy and expensive study, in which the likelihood of any clear-cut results would be exquisitely sensitive to the maintenance of inimical behavior in a large control population? The question was not a simple one, and during the often-heated debates that took place within the National Cancer Advisory Board, memories of Tuskegee were evoked on more than one occasion.

These examples address only a few of the many challenging questions that the collected papers raise. Moreover, given the inevitable changes that will be forthcoming from reform of our health care delivery and reimbursement systems, as well as from the remarkable pace of scientific advancement in biomedicine, many of these moral-ethical issues will only become more prominent.

One issue area worth noting deals with financial conflict of interest which is raised in the paper by Brett and Grodin. These authors point out that under-capitated health plans, which promise to become increasingly prevalent over the next several years, the incentives for physicians are explicitly to underutilize resources since their personal compensation pools are typically at risk in such schemes. Although excessive or inappropriate use of medical resources is a central feature of our present health care financial crisis, Brett and Grodin emphasize that the foundational premise of capitation, namely that "less is better," may not be necessarily true from the perspective of the ailing patient.

Yet another aspect of financial conflict that is not addressed in this set of papers emerges from the research arena. One of the most astonishing results of the "revolution in biology" through which we are living is the remarkable capacity for rapid commercialization of intellectual property that can arise from even the most fundamental lines of biomedical research. Thus, recombinant DNA technology allows the isolation, characterization, and commercial development of myriad exciting new molecules, many with potentially powerful (and lucrative) pharmacological properties. The commercialization process, which is fueled in our society by venture capital, almost always requires that the physician/scientist/inventor "buy into" the business venture and continue to provide close scientific and clinical guidance to the technology transfer that underlies the commercialization process. Ultimately, if the venture is successful, one or more products will be developed and will have to traverse the full gauntlet of clinical trials required to document the safety and efficacy necessary for approval by the Food and Drug Administration (FDA).

In recent years, the NIH, the National Science Foundation, and the FDA, as well as the Congress, have become increasingly concerned about the vexing situations of potential conflict that can arise when physician/scientist/inventors, with substantial financial interests riding on the outcomes, are pivotal participants in the scientific studies and evaluations of products that are required for ultimate approval for marketing. There is still no consensus within the executive and legislative branches of the federal government, nor within the scientific community as to how best to manage such potential conflicts without at the same time dampening scientific creativity and stifling technology transfer. The array of profound moral and ethical conundrums with which we will be confronted can only become more prominent as medical practice and biomedical science continue to break new ground, and "experimentation" on human subjects becomes ever more challenging.

Finally, no commentary concerned with the ethical and moral principles of research on human subjects can be complete without giving at least passing notice to the awesome implications of the national Human Genome Mapping Project, with its extraordinary potential to illuminate the most intimate details of the genetic constitutions of individuals, and thus, their frailties and susceptibility to disease. How will those insights be used most effectively and equitably to mitigate human morbidity and mortality? How will that information be accessed to deal with the often-conflicting demands of society's presumptive right to know and the individual's right to privacy? How will this remarkable stock of important new knowledge be optimally managed to ensure respect for human dignity and conformance with the fundamental ethical precept of autonomy?

CHAPTER X

Ethical Challenges in the Use of Genetic Information

ABSTRACTS AND EXCERPTS

■ Annas GJ. Setting standards for the use of DNA-typing results in the courtroom—the state of the art. *N Engl J Med.* 1992;326:1641-1644.

Abstracted from information appearing in *NEJM*. Reprinted with permission of the *New England Journal of Medicine*.

DNA typing, sometimes called DNA fingerprinting or profiling, has been the focus of heated exchanges in courtrooms, the popular press, and scientific journals. It is a powerful law-enforcement weapon, especially in cases of rape, because it has the potential to exonerate a suspect or to place him at the scene of a crime. . . . When should judges permit evidence from DNA typing to go to the jury, and what part should the medical and scientific literature play in this decision?

Continuing disputes in the nation's courtrooms about the validity and reliability of DNA typing, the methodologic standards to be applied, and the interpretation of population statistics led to a study of the issue by the National Research Council of the National Academy of Sciences.

Several lessons can be drawn from the hasty attempts to introduce the results of DNA typing into the courtroom. The obvious one is that it is more appropriate, and certainly more reliable, to resolve scientific controversies in scientific journals and by means of multidisciplinary scientific committees before they are brought to the courtroom. Attempting to resolve such questions as was initially done in the case of DNA typing effectively requires judges and juries to be arbiters of scientific debates, and at the same time it at least partly converts scientific journals into forums for legal debates on evidentiary standards in the courtroom. The danger for science is probably much more real than the danger in the courtroom, where the judge's instructions, cross-examination, testimony by defense experts, and the appeals process usually prevent grave errors, because actions that might seem reasonable in an adversarial legal process could undermine the more objective scientific process.

The parallel lessons for medicine are equally obvious. . . . appropriate studies of accuracy, efficacy, and safety should be published in peer-reviewed medical journals, and professional societies should take positions on the merits of the new techniques according to their views of sound medical practice, not their views of evidentiary rules or courtroom practices. With such peer review and consensus, the courts can turn to professional literature and professional societies for reliable guidance about the "standard of care."

. . . although DNA-typing evidence may be admissible when the scientists conclude it is generally acceptable, the weight to be given to such evidence in determining guilt or innocence in particular cases is a matter for the jury to decide. Similarly, even after genetic tests are determined to be "standard care" to the extent that they should be routinely offered to patients, the decisions of whether to have the test and what use to make of the information should be left up to the patient.

■ Council on Ethical and Judicial Affairs, American Medical Association. Use of genetic testing by employers. *JAMA.* 1991;266:1827-1830.

Potential applications of information gained from the human genome project extend well beyond the setting of medical care. Employers, insurers, and law enforcement agencies all will have uses for genetic-testing techniques. In many cases, these uses will provide important social benefits. DNA fingerprinting can establish with greater certainty the identity of a criminal; it can also exonerate the innocent defendant. However, our experiences with genetic and other medical testing suggest that abuses may occur. Some companies may have restricted employment opportunities for individuals who carry the sickle cell trait, even though no scientific basis for the restrictions existed. In addition, employment discrimination has occurred repeatedly against individuals because of their medical problems. Previously, irrational fears led employers to deny jobs to patients with cancer or epilepsy. Individuals infected with the human immunodeficiency virus continue to be victims of employment discrimination.

This report will propose guidelines to help physicians assess when their participation in genetic testing by employers is appropriate and does not result in unwarranted discrimination against individuals with genetic abnormalities.

■ Fletcher JC, Anderson WF. Germ-line gene therapy: a new stage of debate. *Law, Medicine and Health Care.* 1992;20:26-39.

Reprinted with permission of the American Society of Law & Medicine

Ethical debate on human germ-line gene therapy is in a new stage. After an era when only individual convictions could be examined, technology is on a threshold of real possibilities. Germ-line gene therapy can conceivably be carried out in either of two practical ways: 1) insertion of a gene into a pre-embryo, which is the subject of this paper, or 2) insertion of a gene into the germ cells of an individual.

Transgenic animal research and pre-implantation embryo diagnosis have implications for human embryonic germ-line experiments to correct single gene disorders. When would such experiments be feasible and ethically acceptable? If further animal research supports it, we argue for a moral obligation to learn if human germ-line experiments are feasible and safe to attempt. The obligation is grounded in several social-ethical principles that lead society and researchers to set goals for studies that promise to relieve and to prevent human suffering and premature death. These principles also shape the practices and restrictions of biomedical research.

Two concurrent processes now need to occur. First, prospects for human germ-line therapy need to be explored in a national forum, in the light of scientific facts and various ethical perspectives. Second, federally-supported research activities that currently have a higher ethical and social priority than human germ-line research need to be reexamined. Some research activities involving the human embryo, fetus, and fetal tissue for transplants now have more immediate promise than germ-line experiments to lead to relief or prevention of suffering caused by genetic disorders and cancer. Obstacles to both types of research need replacement with a coherent set of public policies to permit and oversee federally-supported activities in these areas. This paper traces early ethical debate on this topic, describes a new stage of the debate, presents an ethical argument that could support the first pre-embryo experiments, and discusses the comparative ethical and social priorities of research in germ-line gene therapy and other research activities.

■ **Gostin L. Genetic discrimination: the use of genetically based diagnostic and prognostic tests by employers and insurers. *American J of Law and Med.* 1991;17:109-144.**

Reprinted with permission of the *American Journal of Law and Medicine*.

Genetic discrimination is detrimental to public health programs, as well as to society generally. Advances in genetic testing and screening, accelerated and prompted by the Human Genome Initiative, increase society's ability to detect and monitor chromosomal differences. These technologies and their resulting genomic data will enhance medical science, but may also encourage discrimination. Although few employers or insurers currently utilize genetic screening, testing or data, rising employee benefit costs and market forces create powerful incentives for usage.

Current municipal, state and federal laws, including the Americans with Disabilities Act (ADA), may not sufficiently protect employees and insureds from genetic discrimination. While municipal and state protections should not be overlooked, the ADA's sweeping scope may currently provide the most comprehensive safeguard. Federal laws banning discrimination on the basis of race or sex might also successfully redress some forms of genetic discrimination. Genetic technologies' advent necessitates efforts to rectify state and federal statutory coverage gaps, strictly regulate employers and produce comprehensive guidelines regarding its use.

■ **Juengst ET. Priorities in professional ethics and social policy for human genetics. *JAMA.* 1991;266:1835-1836.**

There are two reasons genetic testing by employers is an important matter for professional and public deliberation, even without an explosion in its practice. The first reason is pedagogical; the second, practical.

For students of professional ethical and social policy questions in human genetics, the significance of workplace genetic screening lies in the value choices it raises as much as in its urgency as a potential social problem. As the report of the Council of Ethical and Judicial Affairs shows, thinking about exclusionary genetic testing by employers underscores three sets of professional and public choices about the use of genetic information: choices about controlling the societal diffusion of genetic testing, protecting the privacy of genetic information, and reducing the risks of genetic discrimination. These same choices, in less dramatic form, confront other uses of genetic testing as well. In fact, it is the heuristic ability of the workplace scenario to illuminate the issues involved in other, more immediate uses of genetic testing that makes its analysis valuable. Collectively, the concerns it highlights provide an agenda for professional ethics and social policy making in human genetics that can help anticipate the advances in clinical genetic testing now on the horizon.

From this perspective, the real challenge of preparing for the responsible use of new human genetic information is to move our discussions beyond (or back from) the heuristic case of workplace testing, to examine each of the three sets as they emerge in the setting of clinical care.

■ Murray TH. Ethical issues in human genome research. *FASEB J.* 1991;5:55-60.

Reprinted with permission of *The FASEB Journal.*

In addition to provocative questions about science policy, research on the human genome will generate important ethical questions in at least three categories. First, the possibility of greatly increased genetic information about individuals and populations will require choices to be made about what that information should be and about who should control the generation and dissemination of genetic information. Presymptomatic testing, carrier screening, workplace genetic screening, and testing by insurance companies pose significant ethical problems. Second, the burgeoning ability to manipulate human genotypes and phenotypes raises a number of important ethical questions. Third, increasing knowledge about genetic contributions to ethically and politically significant traits and behaviors will challenge our self-understanding and social institutions.

The point here is not that we should ignore the influence of genetics on human affairs. Scientists should be the last people to abandon evidence in favor of sentimental, comforting illusion. Lucidity demands that we confront the truth as it is. Rather, we must learn not to overinterpret what we find. We must learn how to communicate effectively among ourselves and with the public about the limits of our knowledge.

Last, we must acknowledge the limited ethical and political significance of our genetic knowledge. When the founders of the United States wrote that all men (all people) are created equal, they did not mean this as a statement of biological fact, but as an ethical, legal, and political proclamation: before the collectivity of the state, all persons must be regarded as equal—each due equal respect, equal liberty, and equal protection, among other fundamental rights. The sciences of inequality, with genetics at the forefront, will force us to reinterpret what equal treatment and equal regard mean in an enormous range of contexts. But they need not threaten the ethical core of that commitment.

■ National Research Council. *DNA Technology in Forensic Science.* Washington, D.C.: National Academy Press; 1992.

Reprinted with permission of the National Academy Press.

Characterization, or "typing," of deoxyribonucleic acid (DNA) for purposes of criminal investigation can be thought of as an extension of the forensic typing of blood that has been common for more than 50 years; it is actually an extension from the typing of proteins that are coded for by DNA to the typing of DNA itself.

DNA typing has great potential benefits for criminal and civil justice; however, because of the possibilities for its misuse or abuse, important questions have been raised about reliability, validity, and confidentiality. . . . the Committee on DNA Technology in Forensic Science was formed . . . to address the general applicability and appropriateness of the use of DNA technology in forensic science, the need to develop standards for data collection and analysis, aspects of the technology, management of DNA typing data, and legal, societal, and ethical issues surrounding DNA typing. The techniques of DNA typing are fruits of the revolution in molecular biology that is yielding an explosion of information about human genetics. The highly personal and sensitive information that can be generated by DNA typing requires strict confidentiality and careful attention to the security of data.

Before any particular DNA typing method is used for forensic purposes, precise and scientifically reliable procedures . . . must be established. It is meaningless to speak of the reliability of DNA typing in general—i.e., without specifying a particular method.

Critics and supporters of the forensic uses of DNA typing agree that there is a lack of standardization of practices and a lack of uniformly accepted methods for quality assurance. The deficiencies are due largely to the rapid emergence of DNA typing and its introduction in the United States through the private sector.

Although standardization of forensic practice is difficult because of the nature of the samples, DNA typing is such a powerful and complex technology that some degree of standardization is necessary to ensure high standards.

Confidentiality and security of DNA-related information are especially important and difficult issues, because we are in the midst of two extraordinary technological revolutions that show no signs of abating: in molecular biology, which is yielding an explosion of information about human genetics, and in computer technology, which is moving toward national and international networks connecting growing information resources.

In the future, if pilot studies confirm its value, a national DNA profile databank should be created that contains information on felons convicted of particular violent crimes.

Courts should take judicial notice of three scientific underpinnings of DNA typing:

> The study of DNA polymorphisms can, in principle, provide a reliable method for comparing samples.

> Each person's DNA is unique (except that of identical twins), although the actual discriminatory power of any particular DNA test will depend on the sites of DNA variation examined.

> The current laboratory procedure for detecting DNA variation . . . is fundamentally sound, although the validity of any particular implementation of the basic procedure will depend on proper characterization of the reproducibility of the system (e.g., measurement variation) and inclusion of all necessary scientific controls.

In the forensic context as in the medical setting, DNA information is personal, and a person's privacy and need for confidentiality should be respected. The release of DNA information on a criminal population without the subjects' permission for purposes other than law enforcement should be considered a misuse of the information, and legal sanctions should be established to deter the unauthorized dissemination or procurement of DNA information that was obtained for forensic purposes.

■ Nelkin D, Tancredi L. Classify and control: genetic information in the schools. *American J of Law and Med.* 1991;17:51-73.

Reprinted with permission of the *American Journal of Law and Medicine.*

This paper addresses and assesses the impact of genetic assumptions on educational practice. In part II, we review recent genetic advances that bear on educational issues and their diffusion into popular culture. Even though sophisticated genetic testing and screening techniques are still limited to experimental investigation, they provide theoretical models that explain complex human behavior—learning disabilities and behavioral problems—in simple biological terms. Part III focuses on the appeal of genetic explanations in light of the institutional imperatives in education. In part IV, we focus on the application of such explanations through biological tests. Part V analyzes the intrinsic difficulties in interpreting genetic information, and Part VI analyzes the social consequences of genetic assumptions for both students and schools. Legal issues implicated by genetic testing are discussed in Part VII.

Schools have long differentiated and classified students through diagnostic and evaluative tests. Detailed and sensitive information about individual children—their genetic makeup, predisposition to violence and mental illness, brain structure and susceptibility to disease—serves well-recognized educational needs. It also serves administrative needs, enhancing efficiency and economy in the management of education. Technologies that assess genetic capabilities and reveal biochemical states that "cause" behavior enable educators to predict which children will be slow learners, disruptive, handicapped or difficult in the classroom.

It is not surprising that the educational establishment is receptive to biological explanations of student behavior. But this model also poses problems within the school system. The most obvious problem is inherent in any form of educational classification, namely labeling and stigmatizing students. Biological classifications can exacerbate the effects of labeling because they imply that the individual, lacking control over behavior, is faced with a permanent and immutable disability. While such explanations remove behavior problems from moral disapproval, they also reduce expectations of those students.

By assuming that biological deficits underlie all learning and behavioral problems, diagnostic techniques have directed attention away from the importance of social interaction in shaping behavior, further mystifying our understanding of learning difficulties.

■ Roberts RJ. The societal impact of DNA fingerprint data. *Accountability in Research.* 1992;2:87-92.

Few scientific techniques have captured the public imagination more than the technique of DNA fingerprinting. When Alec Jeffries first suggested that polymorphic loci in human DNA could be used for identification purposes he can scarcely have realized the furor and debate that would ensue. What began as a straightforward technique to determine relationships among newly arrived immigrants in England soon found its way into the investigation of criminal activities.

There are many issues of data integrity associated with DNA fingerprinting. First and foremost is the quality of the original Southern blot that is to be interpreted by the forensic scientist. Lots of things can go wrong if sloppy techniques are practiced and there are certain inherent difficulties when dealing with forensic samples.

At the present time almost everyone connected with the DNA fingerprinting business as well as those scientists who have thought about it deeply are in agreement that the basic experimental methodology to produce the data is appropriate and reliable. In the U.S.A. it seems likely that appropriate guidelines for making DNA fingerprints by RFLP [Restriction Length Polymorphism] technology will soon be in place. Data integrity has occasionally been an issue in court, but for the most part good data can readily be distinguished from bad data even by non-experts. More controversial, however, is the interpretation of the data in terms of the statistics of matching. If humans were a random breeding population the statistics would be rather easy. However, they are not. For geographic, cultural, racial, religious or other reasons one often finds small subpopulations developing in which gene frequencies can be very skewed. This can greatly complicate our ability to estimate the real probabilities of matching.

By far the most difficult issue to deal with in the forensic setting concerns the quality of the data that should be viewed as acceptable. From a purely scientific viewpoint one would like to see perfect data or at least as good as can be produced routinely in a research laboratory. However, the two situations are very different.

. . . while no one would want to see really awful data accepted into evidence, it is equally unfair to insist that the data must be perfect every time. Neither science, justice nor society are well-served by such rigorous demands.

. . . it is imperative that regulations concerning the generation of DNA fingerprint data and its subsequent interpretation should be laid out by a panel of scientists, aided by lawyers and other individuals who will have to deal with the results of the regulations.

In conclusion, the forensic use of DNA fingerprinting is one area where scientific data meets society head on. The data must be reliable, but not necessarily perfect. Scientists presenting and interpreting it have special responsibilities to ensure that the science is done properly and that it is reported fairly and accurately. In the normal course of research there are many checks and bounds that limit the damage that can be done by faulty data collection and interpretation. Often those same checks and bounds cannot be guaranteed when forensic evidence is involved. While this should not exclude the use of DNA evidence it should make the scientists producing and interpreting it very cautious and critical. For in addition to the defendant, science and scientific methods are themselves on trial.

■ **Zimmerman BK. Human germ-line therapy: the case for its development and use. *J Med Philos.* 1991;16:593-612.**

The rationale for pursuing the development and use of germ-line selection and modification techniques is examined in this essay. The argument is put forth that it is the moral obligation of the medical profession to make available to the public any technology that can cure or prevent pathology leading to death and disability, in both the present and future generations. Society should pursue the development of strategies for preventing or correcting, at the germ-line level, genetic features that will lead to, or enhance, pathological conditions. Because prenatal screening and even early embryo screening and selection can prevent only a subset of known genetic disorders, direct genetic intervention is the *only* way in which certain couples can exercise their rights to reproductive health.

Direct genetic manipulation of the pre-embryo should be carried out only if the methods used ensure with a very high probability that (a) a specific correction of a defective gene will be made; (b) the procedure will not introduce any genetic errors or new genetic material that could have unpredictable effects in subsequent generations; and (c) that such procedures include a check to ensure that the procedure has been carried out as intended, before allowing a pregnancy to proceed.

One may conclude that, at this time, provided the technical reliability of the procedures can be assured as stated above, there is no compelling reason not to proceed with the development and use of such methods, beginning with applications to prevent severe genetic pathology.

. . . policies that may govern applications of germ-line methods that go beyond the prevention of pathology require a thorough evaluation by society of criteria that transcend the traditional considerations of principles of individual autonomy, the rights and responsibilities of individuals, and distributive justice.

COMMENTARY

Jack D. Barchas and Isaac D. Barchas

Although the development of techniques for analyzing and manipulating genetic information poses important ethical questions for society, let us be clear: genetic ethics is not about Jurassic Park. Rather, for the foreseeable future, issues of genetic ethics will center around individual medical cases. Using genetic information to diagnose and treat disease is already proving of great benefit to doctors and patients. At this time, the most serious ethical issues seem to involve the dissemination of this information to institutions that may not share the physician's concern for the individual's well-being. This commentary addresses the use of genetic information in the contexts both of the doctor-patient relationship and in the context of the relationship between the patient and a third party.

The use of genetic information in medical therapy often provides clear benefits to individuals. Many, if not most, of these therapies present few ethical problems and have enormous potential to alleviate catastrophic human suffering. Some of these genetic therapies actually attempt to remedy or ameliorate diseases caused by genetic defects. Worldwide efforts to use the tools of molecular genetics for cystic fibrosis is one such example.

Perhaps the most promising therapeutic use of genetic information, however, will be in the treatment of diseases that may not have a genetic origin, such as Parkinson's disease and cancer. Parkinson's disease may be due to unknown viral or environmental toxins, or to toxins generated by the brain by mechanisms not yet understood. Yet methods are being developed to utilize molecular genetic approaches for treatment. The introduction of genes into the brain using methods such as viral vectors for nerve growth factors or to replace neuroregulators are examples of the use of gene therapy to treat an illness that may not have an origin that is primarily genetic. Similarly, methods are being developed to introduce genetic information into brain tumors that could stop their growth, regardless of their originating cause.

These examples of the pharmaceutical use of genetic information are viewed as positive developments by most people. Appropriately more controversial, although practically still some time in the future, are issues related to directed alteration of the germ line. Even most advocates of gene therapy view such use of genetic information as profoundly dangerous. Eugenics directed at humans is inimical to almost all significant ethical traditions. It also dramatically fails the test of our historical memory. The dangers of eugenically motivated germ line "therapies"—say, to increase intelligence—place the use of truly therapeutic germ line manipulation—say, to prevent sickle-cell anemia—in an ethically ambiguous position. Indeed, the complexity of genetic information is such that the physiological effects of gene expression may be multiple and diffuse, further complicating the therapeutic use of germ line therapies.

However, we must keep in mind that germ line therapies represent only one of the medically significant uses of genetic information. Most of the other uses of this information, such as pharmacological uses, present fewer ethical problems. Ironically, though, it is the very existence of this information, rather than its medical use, that may present the most potent and practical ethical issues. The existence of genetic information itself raises the issues of privacy and access that lie at the heart of much of the debate on this topic.

Many components of the social system want access to an individual's medical information, of which genetic information will surely soon be a routine part. And, indeed, many people and institutions have some sort of legitimate claim on that information: patients, doctors, relatives, insurers, employers, and government. Clearly, the interests of these actors may conflict, perhaps dramatically, in ways too numerous to mention here.

Concerning these issues of access and testing, ethicists and policy makers should ask whether genetic information is different in kind from other medical information. Surely the quantity of information contained on the genome is vast. Yet, practically, is there a qualitative difference between knowing that a patient has a genetic predisposition to heart disease and the conventionally obtained information that the patient has an extraordinarily high cholesterol level? Moreover, genetic information, though frequently diagnostically useful, is often difficult to manage statistically. The etiologies of many diseases with a genetic component are often diffuse and difficult to pin down, as they frequently involve the expression of multiple genes and/or the interaction of genetic and environmental factors.

Perhaps one way to view the ethical issues surrounding the availability of genetic information would be to treat it as comparable to the other forms of information that are already widely available, such as medical information, financial information, and biographical information. The question is: do current legal structures adequately manage these forms of information—and, by extension, can they balance the interests of the parties concerned with genetic information? Viewing genetic information in this manner, as part of a continuum of information rather than as a unique information product that demands unique safeguards, would allow policy makers to employ existing paradigms to guide its use.

Indeed, if the debates about genetic ethics are not to dissolve into casuistry, drawing upon our society's rich legal and social heritage of information management seems to be imperative.

Clearly, access to genetic information raises serious issues: What is informed consent in the providing of samples? How will the data be interpreted? To what extent is a genetic disposition the same as the occurrence of a metabolic process? What other factors are at work in the development of a genetic predisposition? Who will be told? What privacy protection does the individual have? Will the information be used to prevent options for the individual to which he or she would otherwise be entitled?

To a greater or lesser degree, all of these questions are raised by other types of information as well. As banal as it may seem to say so, information as devastating for individuals and their future options can be obtained in a credit check. Genetic information, unique as it may be to the individual, is not unique in the ethical and policy questions it raises. Genetic information, like many other sorts of information, must be integrated into a system of law that both protects the individual about whom the information in generated and satisfies other parties with legitimate interests in that information.

COMMENTARY

Roger J. Bulger

The 10 articles and essays in this chapter present a nice sampling of the wide array of societal issues raised by the new genetics. Deoxyribonucleic acid (DNA) was discovered just 50 years ago; the double helix model was discovered and promulgated by Watson and Crick 40 years ago. The pace of basic science progress in genetics over the past four decades has increased exponentially, and the time separating basic from applied science in genetics has truncated such that today's molecular biologist may become next week's biotechnology mogul.

In the decade of the 1980s, an entirely new biotechnology industry was created and established, which was built on DNA technology. This achievement has been largely American and is attributed to a non-obstructive governmental policy in combination with highly effective relationships between academe and business. These relationships have ensured that technology reaches the bedside and have spawned numerous new companies. Taken in the aggregate, the multiplicity of biotechnology companies is approximately equal in size to the largest single pharmaceutical corporation.

Now, the human genome project in the United States and similar efforts in Europe promise to hasten the evolution of genetic diagnostics, therapeutics, and preventive interventions. In fact, some observers point out that for some time to come we shall be in the frustrating period of being able to diagnose genetic abnormalities without having a therapeutic or corrective response in hand. Hardly a week goes by without the announcement that a precise genetic abnormality has been identified which is associated with a particular disease. Most recently, the finding of a genetic defect in patients with amyotrophic lateral sclerosis (ALS) or Lou Gehrig's disease was broadcast by the media. Some articles seemed to promise a short time frame until effective therapy is available. But buried deep in these stories was the fact that the genetic defect was found in only a portion of ALS patients. We as a society are ripe for overpromise and are being set up for major disappointments down the road.

Our growing capacity to use genetics to diagnose, to classify or categorize, or to identify abnormalities raises issues that are dealt with in several of the articles and papers. Our ability to identify Huntington's disease in many people well before they become symptomatic is a dramatic example that illustrates the problems that can arise from our new knowledge and discoveries. These people may go without signs or symptoms of the disease and live to their fourth or fifth decade, only to decline over a few short years to meet a certain death. The ability to make such diagnoses and prognoses has led to many ethical questions about the use of such genetic tests to make decisions about employment or insurance eligibility. Although most of us agree that it is not right to use such tests for these purposes, it is apparently true that even the much-heralded Americans with Disabilities Act does not seem to close all the loopholes open to employers and health insurers to discriminate or refuse coverage.

While most of the debate centers on the use of this information to discriminate against patients, it is also possible that patients could misuse the information for their own gain. A Huntington's patient, asymptomatic but certain of the diagnosis, could purchase large amounts of life insurance.

The prospect of an identifiable genetic abnormality or abnormalities associated with Alzheimer's disease raises new specters. In California, it is the doctor's responsibility to report the diagnosis of Alzheimer's disease to the state. If a person is in an automobile accident and is found to have Alzheimer's, and if the physician has not reported it, the physician is held responsible for the accident. On the other hand, if the doctor reports the patient, then the patient will lose his or her driver's license.

The high profile that genetic diagnostics and therapeutics have attained in the public's mind easily leads to extensive over-reliance upon the test or intervention. DNA finger printing, for example, has rapidly gained the trust of the public, leaving little room for understanding that these tests are not perfect.

The therapeutic germline interventions of Steven Rosenberg in 1990 and French Andersen in 1992 have brought another sort of issue to the foreground, that of cost and equity. The impact of the enormous cost of gene therapy for one person is bound to raise equity questions with regard to those people who cannot get that treatment or with regard to some other treatment that was forced off the list of basic benefits for economic reasons. If and when a germline intervention comes along for a disease as widespread, for example, as diabetes, the prospect would become imminent of a multi-billion dollar add-on to the national health care bill, thus eventually raising difficult decisions about prioritization and resource allocation.

Just as basic thermonuclear science and its applied counterpart had profound national societal implications, so too molecular genetics has highlighted the moral, legal, and ethical impact of science on our population. All this argues ever more strongly for a health care work force which is more sophisticated than our current one in philosophy, political science, economics, bioethics, and the law.

The power of genetics to shape social policy and influence our society may soon help end the practice of experience-rating in the insurance industry, as our population learns that companies under experience-rating will segment the population, raking off those with the best genes and offering them the lowest prices. That degree of segmentation or societal fragmentation is unacceptable. The total burden of illness must be spread among the entire population; charging each person equally for health insurance (or "community rating") must become the norm.

CHAPTER XI

Effects of Biomedical Research on Patient Care

ABSTRACTS AND EXCERPTS

■ **Annas GJ. The human genome project as social policy: implications for clinical medicine. *Bulletin of the NY Academy of Medicine.* 1992;68:126-134.**

Reprinted with permission, courtesy of the New York Academy of Medicine.

I shall review three areas in clinical genetics where the genome project will have an impact. But the first and most important point I want to make is that it is not the human genome project that produced these problems. The genome project may make them more immediate and critical by providing us more products that can be used in clinical medicine, but it did not create these basic problems.

It may in fact be true, as Norton Zinder has argued, that the genome project is not skewing molecular biology research. It is not true, however, that the genome project is not skewing bioethics research. At 3% of the budget, funding could be $90 million over 15 years. This is more money than has ever been spent on bioethics in the United States. And even the annual budget right now is more money than is being spent on all the other bioethical issues put together. So if you want to talk about distortion of activities, one likely distortion is in the area of bioethics. On the other hand, the genome project raises almost all of the fundamental issues in bioethics.

. . . the first central issue is whether or not a concentration on genetics will lead our society to undervalue the influence of the environment and to overvalue the influence of genetics.

The second issue get us more directly into clinical genetics, the issue of genetic screening and counseling.

The ultimate issue, of course, is who we screen, when we screen them, what we screen for, and who makes the decision about what to do with the information that is gained by screening?

It is now possible to counsel and to screen people for only a handful of specific genetic diseases. But once we get dozens or hundreds of genetic conditions that people can be screened for it will then become impossible, literally, to get informed consent for each one and to do meaningful counseling for each one prior to screening. The question will then be whether one can develop some kind of "generic" genetic screening and counseling.

Finally, let me just say a few words about therapy, since we all say that the ultimate goal of all this research is to develop new human health and disease insights that could, hopefully, lead to treatment.

The long debate about somatic cell gene experimentation and therapy in the United States is more or less resolved. The model that is being used is, I think appropriately so, the general model of treating any illness. Treating an illness at the somatic cell level is seen as substantially the same as giving a drug, or at least like transplantation. The key is again to resolve the ethical and legal issues in advance. An experiment is ethical or not at the time that it is performed, not in retrospect.

. . . even though people like to make the argument that we are not going to enhance characteristics, that is the only thing that makes any sense to do with the embryos. To make a bigger mouse, a smarter kid, a bigger kid, or whatever. [sic] We say that we're not going to do that because we can draw the line between disease and enhancement I would like someone to show me that line. That line is probably impossible to draw if we go into the area of germ-line gene therapy. It thus seems to me that the major danger we run is the possibility of creating not an underclass, but an overclass. The rich will not only be richer than you and I, they will be the ones who will be able to take advantage of germ-line gene therapy to engineer their kids in ways we haven't thought of yet.

In conclusion and summary, let me say that my guess is that, as with Apollo, in which the main product turned out to be the photograph of the earth and the beginning of environmental awareness on this planet, we may not yet know what the main product of the human genome project will be. . . . autonomy and respect for individual choice (self-determination), although it is under tremendous attack by the new genetics, must, I think, remain the cornerstones of clinical genetic medicine. The challenge is real, and dedicated funding for ethical, legal, and social issues, as well as meaningful public debate is a necessary, though not sufficient, component of the human genome project in America.

■ Baum BJ. Has modern biology entered the mouth? The clinical impact of biological research. *Journal of Dental Education.* 1991;55:299-303.

Reprinted with permission of the *Journal of Dental Education.*

I'd like to address, through this essay, whether advances in biological research have had any significant clinical impact on dentistry and what this might mean for the future.

I honestly don't think biologists, in particular oral biologists such as myself, have had a substantive clinical impact on dentistry. I believe oral biologists have made enormous research progress and have given the scientific community and dental profession many meaningful contributions over the past 15 years. But the impact of modern biology has scarcely been felt by the dental educator or practitioner. Why is this so?

The notion that biological research is relevant to dentistry, indeed that it will change dentistry, is simply not fostered in our schools.

I think that the eventual clinical impact of biological research will be to change the nature of dentistry.

Dentistry (and therefore oral health care) is now in a transition period. It can sit back and let external forces completely influence the direction it takes. Alternatively, dentistry can be a participant in its own development and, as a corollary, markedly improve oral health care for Americans.

. . . oral biologists cannot lead dentistry through this transition period. They must (and I believe will) only supply some tools. The leadership and greater responsibility lies with dental educators (oral biologist or not). Progress in biology and medicine is rapid and dental education is not keeping pace. This situation cannot, and should not, continue. Dental educators need to change dental education, release it from its lethargy, and allow students to be exposed to the practical advances of biomedical research, not just to basic science lectures. . . . Oral biologists must help educators bring biological and biomedical advances into the training of future dentists in a meaningful way. Universities must allow these changes to take place and organized dentistry (accrediting and licensing agencies) must cooperate with these endeavors. Flexibility and innovation are needed to train the transitional dentist. Irrespective of dentistry's response, I have no doubt that within 25 years, the impact of modern biology on dentistry will be evident and that it will lead to a re-definition of the profession.

■ Council on Ethical and Judicial Affairs, American Medical Association. Gender disparities in clinical decision making. *JAMA*. 1991;266:559-562.

Recent evidence has raised concerns that women are disadvantaged because of inadequate attention to the research, diagnosis, and treatment of women's health care problems. In 1985, the US Public Health Services' Task Force on Women's Health Issues reported that the lack of research data on women limited understanding of women's health needs.

Physicians should examine their practices and attitudes for the influence of social or cultural biases that could affect medical care. Physicians must ensure that gender is not used inappropriately as a consideration in clinical decision making. Assessments of need based on presumptions about the relative worth of certain social roles must be avoided. Procedures and techniques that preclude or minimize the possibility of gender bias should be developed and implemented. A gender-neutral determination for kidney transplant eligibility should be used.

More medical research on women's health and women's health problems should be pursued. Results of medical testing done solely on men should not be generalized to women without evidence that results can be applied safely and effectively to both sexes. Research on health problems that affect both sexes should include male and female subjects. Sound medical and scientific reasons should be required for excluding women from medical tests and studies, such as that the proposed research does not or would not affect the health of women. An obvious example would be research on prostatic cancer. Also, further research into the possible causes of gender disparities should be conducted. The extent to which physician-patient interactions may be influenced by cultural and social conceptions of gender should be ascertained.

Finally, awareness of and responsiveness to sociocultural factors that could lead to gender disparities may be enhanced by increasing the number of female physicians in leadership roles and other positions of authority in teaching, research, and the practice of medicine.

■ **Levine C, Stein GL. What's in a name? The policy implications of the CDC definition of AIDS.** *Law, Medicine and Health Care.* **1991;19:278-290.**

Reprinted with permission of the American Society of Law & Medicine

Disease classification systems and surveillance definitions are ordinarily tools for medical professionals, not matters for political debate and patient advocacy.

The Centers for Disease Control's (CDC) case definition of AIDS is used by public health officials, researchers, clinicians, hospital administrators, disability specialists, insurance administrators, health economists, legislators, social workers, policy makers, and the media. It has influenced the way the HIV epidemic is perceived, managed, and funded.

It is not surprising, then, that the CDC definition of AIDS and its proposed revision is currently the subject of intense scrutiny. The case definition has transcended epidemiology to become a symbol for the inadequacies of the U.S. government's response to the HIV epidemic, and a particular symbol for the failure to address the needs of HIV-infected women.

In this broad context, this paper has two straightforward and limited intentions: first, to distinguish the primary purpose of the CDC's surveillance definition from the ancillary uses that it triggers in entitlements and benefits, funding formulas, clinical research, medical care, and calculations of the costs of health care and social services; and second, to offer some recommendations for action and areas for further study. There are two overarching questions. First, is the CDC definition fulfilling its primary epidemiological purpose? Second, are the ancillary uses of this surveillance tool appropriate?

The existence of several different systems that describe HIV and AIDS—two within the CDC itself—has led to confusion and uncertainty.

At a minimum, it appears that something of importance has been missed in surveillance based on the current definition—primarily diseases unique to women.

Although the CDC's various case definitions were developed primarily for surveillance activities, these definitions have become the diagnostic standard used by other federal, state, and local agencies to determine eligibility for entitlements and benefits. This has had a significant impact, both positive and negative.

Changing the CDC definition of AIDS would probably have a mixed impact on private insurance and disability benefits.

Changing the case definition of AIDS might lead to a reallocation of resources. But unless overall allocations are increased, if some area benefits, another loses.

Advocates for revising the CDC definition of AIDS have charged that the current formulation results in poor clinical care because physicians fail to recognize and treat appropriately HIV-related diseases that are not AIDS-defining.

The primary reasons most physicians use the CDC definition are to determine when a case should be reported to local public health authorities or to determine whether a particular patient can be certified as "disabled" to obtain benefits.

The CDC definition has only a loose relationship to the way doctors practice medicine, and as noted, the CDC explicitly denies that the definition should be used to determine clinical care.

On balance, concerns about the CDC's proposal seem to outweigh its advantages. These concerns are primarily the absence of additional specific AIDS-defining conditions, the reliance on laboratory tests that are inaccessible to the populations already undercounted, and the threats to confidentiality from state legislation overriding traditional public health protection of reported names. Until these concerns are addressed, we do not recommend adoption of the CDC proposal.

■ **Meyer BR. Biotechnology and therapeutics: expensive treatments and limited resources. A view from the hospital.** *Clinical Pharmacology & Therapeutics.* **1992;51:359-365.**

Reprinted with permission from Mosby-Year Book, Inc.

The 40 years after World War II witnessed a "revolution" in medical therapeutics.

We are now entering what will be a "second drug revolution.". . . Most of the important new drugs of the next decade will not be simple organic molecules but larger and more complex polypeptide and protein compounds. These compounds offer the opportunity for dramatic changes in therapeutics.

This new generation of pharmaceutical products differs from those of the preceding decade in two very important respects: (1) These new products are more difficult and expensive to develop and produce for clinical use, and (2) these products are emerging at a time when the seemingly unlimited resources devoted to health care research and delivery during the first decades after World War II are no longer available.

The introduction of expensive new products at a time of shrinking resources poses special challenges to clinical pharmacologists and to all physicians concerned with the introduction of new therapies into clinical medicine.

ISSUES FOR DISCUSSION

What are the costs and benefits of the introduction of these new agents?

What surrogate end points are acceptable and valid for clinical trials and when do we need to look at the actual outcomes in question instead of the surrogate?

We must reexamine our policy that all physicians may prescribe any approved drug.

We must reexamine the idea that once a drug is approved for use, it may be routinely prescribed for nonapproved indications.

We must reexamine the idea that the individual physician at the bedside is a source of major therapeutic innovation.

We as a society must begin to reexamine our allocation of resources and analyze the cost of application of these technologies to the clinical context.

The industry of biotechnology must recognize the limited resources that are available and must accept limits on its investment return.

This problem provides a new opportunity for the hospital-based clinical pharmacologist.

COMMENTARY

Thomas Detre

During the past 25 years, more than at any other time in the history of medicine, our knowledge in biological sciences has advanced at a dizzying pace. We have discovered new drugs and chemical entities; and we are on the threshold of using gene transfer for therapeutic purposes. Along with vaccines, gene transfer shows considerable promise for controlling certain cancers, and thus marks our entrance into an entirely new phase of therapeutics.

Both the young middle-aged and middle-aged segments of our population are healthier than ever. Cerebrovascular and cardiovascular diseases are on the decline; thanks to advances in anesthesiology and critical care medicine, we are capable of saving neonates who would not have survived two decades ago. Older patients have a much improved chance to survive surgical procedures, and the old-old—those 80 years of age or older—constitute the fastest growing segment of our population. Our ability to return people to productive work is also unprecedented.

Since sophisticated laboratory tests and novel functional imaging techniques have eliminated most invasive diagnostic methods and a significant percentage of surgical procedures are performed with laparascopic techniques that require brief hospitalization or none at all, the majority of patients are now treated as outpatients. Even though hospital stays in the United States are the shortest in the world, the cost of inpatient care continues to rise because only the most severely ill—those with multiple organ failures, multiple life-threatening injuries, or cancers refractory to "traditional treatments"—are hospitalized.

AIDS, too, contributes to rising health care costs. According to recent estimates, AIDS will require an outlay of $15 billion annually by 1995 in the United States. This tragic illness has, however, taught us important lessons about the role of science in health care.

If it were not for the progress made in molecular biology, the virus (or viruses) responsible for AIDS could not have been identified, and we would be completely powerless to stop the spread of this disease. Observing this catastrophic illness has also confirmed many of our suspicions. Most significant, that the weakening of the immune system, by whatever means it occurs, produces a surge in certain cancers. This finding will improve our understanding of malignant diseases and their management.

Despite the spectacular successes of modern medicine, questions are now being asked about the wisdom of unleashing our expensive armamentarium on those who do not have even the slightest chance of having a reasonable quality of life. Satisfactory answers to these questions are not readily available. Perhaps everybody senses the danger that may arise from taking action for the sake of cost containment; the government will be placed in the position of making decisions about who should live and who should die.

Unexpectedly, prevention, which is touted as the "ultimate" solution to rising health care costs, presents us with the same dilemma. Teaching patients about healthy lifestyles is certainly cost-effective. In the near future, tests derived from molecular biology will enable us to identify people who are at high risk for certain diseases. The need to monitor these people who are likely to be vulnerable throughout their lifetimes, will reduce the use of expensive tertiary care, but will be the source of new expenditures.

The government's efforts to control costs by regulatory procedures are also unlikely to yield the desired results, given our ability to save patients with multiple organ failures, regardless of age. Withholding life-saving treatment, however, is viewed as abhorrent by our society, which is opposed to rationing. Perhaps the only morally defensible approach would be to forgo the use of treatments that are not of definable benefit. Another solution would be to forgo the use of life-saving measures when the likely outcome is survival without reasonable quality of life.

While the populist view is that our society spends too much money on science and technology, the history of medicine is replete with examples of how finding solutions to these complex problems calls for more rather than less science in health care. A concerted, well-planned effort to evaluate the efficacy of diagnostic methods and treatments, replacing what is now in many instances a haphazard approach to care, is an absolute necessity. But, even if practice guidelines based on solid data were available, the use of ineffective and costly methods would continue unabated unless third-party payers (be they the government or private insurers) make reimbursement for diagnostic and treatment procedures contingent on following these guidelines.

COMMENTARY

Donald C. Harrison

Each of the reports abstracted in this chapter describes new technologies, drugs, and scientific definitions that will potentially impact the diagnosis and treatment of human disease. Each raises important considerations in bioethics, public policy for allocating public resources for research and therapy, the basis for the conflict between societal goals and individual expectations, and the influence of these factors on the future of biomedical research. Considerable public policy debate is likely to be generated during the coming decade to find an appropriate balance in each of these areas. It is important for individual patient care and for our society to find a balance which provides support for continuing the "biotechnical and biomedical revolution" of which we are just seeing the dawn. This revolution will have much to do with the quality of life for the human race as we move into the 21st century. My approach will be to outline personal views of some of the scientific and public policy issues raised in these reports.

In my view, the human genome project is one of the most ambitious biomedical projects ever undertaken. However, by using media hype, it has been oversold by the scientists working in genetics and has resulted in diverting funds away from other needy biomedical research projects. It has also been reported that the human genome project competes with funding for delivering medical services to underserved populations. In my view this project provides great promise for the future, and the tradeoff—even though exaggerated by advertising and hype—is still one of the most worthy in which biomedical scientists are involved and should continue to be funded.

The genome project raises many ethical questions, but I will focus on only three. Three to five percent of the budget for this overall project has been allocated for bioethics. This is far more than is spent on bioethics in all other research projects in the United States. Unless there is some fundamental new direction for these studies, my view is that the funds will not be spent wisely. While worthy of study, such issues as whether a human is just a package of genes, or how the genome project will affect doctor-patient relationships, do not demand this kind of support.

Second, the human genome project raises the question of who should be genetically screened, when should screening be made available, who should pay for screening, and what should be the outcome of screening. The appropriate framing of these issues for societal consideration may require considerable resources. There will, of necessity, be legal and constitutional issues as well as clinical research issues, including the impossibility of providing informed consent for each of the screening techniques. My view is that media attention should be focused on this matter primarily to inform the public, so that appropriate representation and general consensus can be developed. Some of the funds allocated for bioethics could be spent in these programs.

The greatest promise for the human genome project is to develop therapy for disease. At present, we have only begun this type of research. I believe the issue of somatic cell gene experimentation has been resolved. Treating an illness by these gene implants is comparable to giving a drug. The future for therapy by these biotechnologies is vast. The major unresolved question is whether germ-line gene experimentation should be carried out and how it should be monitored. It will be possible to provide such therapy in the very near future, and considerable public attention needs to be brought to bear on this issue. It will be difficult to limit the use of biotechnology to make healthier, smarter, and bigger humans. As yet, the limits of the application of biotechnology for these purposes can only be part of human imagination. We must develop a public understanding and consensus on these questions before embarking on the ensuing research.

Since 1985, a considerable body of literature has been published concerning gender disparity in medical research. A preponderance of research in many areas has related to disease in men. More recently it has been suggested that there is a gender difference in the diagnosis and treatment of specific cardiovascular diseases. Review of existing literature confirms with certainty that in specific studies relating to coronary heart disease, women were almost systematically excluded. On the other hand, most studies relating to the utilization of medical services strongly suggests that women receive more health care services overall than do men. Specifically with renal disease and long-term dialysis, the discrepancies that have been reported to favor men can be explained on the basis of dialysis being performed in younger patients, and that a larger percentage of these younger patients with renal failure are men. In coronary heart disease, more attention has been given to the diagnosis and treatment in men because there is a great discrepancy in the number of men developing coronary heart disease in the 40-60-year age group as compared to women. In some cohort groups, this represents values of four to five times as much disease in men.

My overall conclusions from reading the enclosed article and related reports suggest that women have been systematically excluded from certain biomedical research cohorts when the diseases under study are more prominent in males. On the other hand, gender is absolutely necessary for studies on breast cancer, prostatic cancer, and other areas of biology where there is a clear difference between male and female prevalence. Whatever the case, it appears to many to be poorly timed and ill-planned to launch new research ventures that are solely related to gender.

There is no evidence that women have been excluded from a level of service for health care when compared to men. On the other hand, I believe men, because they are more reluctant to visit physicians, receive less medical care overall than women. When compared to women it has not been determined whether this accounts for men's lessened life span.

Recent recommendations by the Centers for Disease Control (CDC) to expand the definition of AIDS to include patients who have specific low levels of T-cells to less than 200 per cubic millimeter of blood have been extensively debated in the literature. Using this definition, the number of individuals who are classified as AIDS victims, as opposed to those with human immunodeficiency virus (HIV)-positive status, is markedly increased. This brings these individuals into the public sector for treatment and resource utilization. This public policy change has been hailed by many as moving toward a more rational policy for managing HIV-positive patients. This particular issue raises many other questions relating to research, clinical care, and therapy for AIDS.

Many have argued that AIDS and the HIV medical problem have received an inordinate amount of attention in research and therapy, as compared to other diseases which involve far more individuals in the U.S. population. The rapid increase of funding for research relating to HIV has, to a large extent, been at the expense of increasing funds for cancer, heart disease, and neuroscience research. In my view, the problem should not be considered competitive, but as the matter now stands, HIV studies have received more than their share of funding from the public sector. Redress of this discrepancy could best be accomplished by increasing the funding for all biomedical research.

The "biomedical revolution," although now in its infancy, is producing many complex polypeptide and protein compounds that will dramatically change therapeutics. This might be entitled "The Second Drug Revolution" and promises therapy for many conditions that have previously been resistant to any therapeutic intervention. Many of these therapies have proven to be extremely expensive.

This factor heightens the questions relating to cost benefit and the rationing of scarce health care resources. Several intensive investigations of cost effectiveness for the polypeptide compounds have been performed and provide equivocal answers.

First, with the synthetic production of erythropoietin, it was clear that many thousands of Americans could benefit from this therapy, especially those patients with low hematocrits and renal failure. While this is a useful drug, its utilization already costs more than $500 million per year. It is also clear that secondary diseases develop due to its long-term use in patients with chronic anemia. These patients may further exacerbate the cost of medical care.

Second, tissue plasminogen activators (tPA) were developed for the treatment of thrombosis in coronary arteries that resulted in acute myocardial infarction. tPA has been studied extensively in comparison with streptokinase as a thrombolytic agent. Recent studies have demonstrated that when given early after acute myocardial infarction, there is equal benefit from the two compounds. However, tPA continues to be widely used although it costs more than 10 times as much per administration as does streptokinase. This raises the question of how physicians can be taught to use more cost-effective forms of therapy in the light of media and medical literature barrages on the effectiveness of such agents as tPA.

Third, major cost effectiveness and ethical issues have been raised by the development of monoclonal antibodies for the treatment of gram-negative sepsis. It has been estimated that for treating a single episode, there is a cost of $3,000 for the agent and, in general, the false-positive rate of 75 percent for clinical use would suggest that successful treatment of a single patient would cost at least $12,000. How this therapy may be used in the future in cost-effective medicine and whether or not it should be rationed (i.e., given only to patients with other life-threatening diseases) is still open to question.

The introduction of each of these new products has demonstrated over-enthusiastic acceptance by the medical profession. In each instance it raises the question, "Is this form of therapy for every individual too costly for the medical care system?"

The specific example cited raises questions which we in the medical profession must answer. Clearly there need to be limits on which physicians prescribe some of the new biotherapeutic compounds. This will require society reexamining the allocation of resources and analyzing the application of these technologies in clinical context. Physicians must play a major role in this reexamination. New start-up companies that produce genetically engineered compounds must be willing to accept less profit on their newly introduced products and less return for investors in such companies. This must occur without unduly restricting the amount of capital available for such new product development.

Finally, in our medical colleges and hospitals we must develop new types of training for physicians who utilize these new therapeutic approaches.

Of the biomedical professions, dentistry has been one of the most resistant to the change produced by the early biomedical revolution. Genetic engineering, molecular biology, and the generation of new therapeutic approaches involving polypeptides and proteins for oral health have not yet been brought into the mainstream of dentistry. It would appear that the oral health of the population could be markedly altered by many of these compounds and concepts. Future therapy that may limit caries will change the total course of dentistry in the next decade. Those involved in dental education will need to appreciate these transitions and involve them in the training of the next generation of dentists. The organized profession, in my view, must make way for such innovations.

Many ethical problems relating to cost-effective therapy are raised by the new biology with which we now have become so accustomed. A major initiative for physicians of the future, particularly those involved in academic medicine, will be to define the issues in terms where public policy can be made. Our public duty will be to bring these therapeutic and diagnostic advances to public attention and scrutiny for societal decisions.

CHAPTER XII

Controversial and Emerging Issues

ABSTRACTS AND EXCERPTS

■ **Annas GJ. Using genes to define motherhood—the California solution. *N Engl J Med.* 1992;326:417-420.**

Abstracted from information appearing in *NEJM*. Reprinted with permission of the *New England Journal of Medicine*.

Sometimes (although not often) new forms of medical technology raise unique legal and social-policy issues that require new laws. In vitro fertilization, followed by the transfer of the embryo to a woman who did not contribute the ovum, is such a technique, because when the child's gestational mother is not the child's genetic mother, society must decide which is the child's legal mother. A California Court of Appeal, the first appellate court anywhere in the world to rule on this issue, decided in late 1991 that genes determine motherhood.

The justices ultimately decided that the genetic mother is the natural mother because "the whole process of human development 'is set in motion by the genes.'" But, of course, the same statement can be made on behalf of the gestational mother. Without her body and her pregnancy, human development would not have continued.

We currently live in an age in which genes are seen, as all the California judges in this case saw them, as the key to human existence. But what then of the large number of women who are capable of carrying a child to term but who cannot produce ova? They now rely on donated ova (rather than gestational surrogacy) to enable them to give birth to children. If the judges are correct, the "natural" mothers of these children are the donors of the ova, not the women who give birth to the children. This conclusion would make current ovum-donation programs unworkable.

It is unfair to criticize the courts too harshly for not arriving at the ultimate solution to this unique and complex question, in which three adults are intimately involved in producing a child to whose development all have contributed biologically and emotionally (if not genetically). Although the court's approach seems both misdirected and unfair, the best solution is not obvious. . . . the reality of this case and others like it is that the child has two mothers, a gestational mother and a genetic mother. Society should acknowledge this biologic fact and take it into account in allocating the rights and responsibilities of parenthood. . . . Public policy must acknowledge the complexity of gamete donation and ultimately take into consideration the best interests of the child.

It will be especially important for physicians to be actively involved as this issue moves from the courts to the state legislatures, which currently have the constitutional authority to enact any laws that are "rational."

■ Beauchamp TL. The moral standing of animals in medical research. *Law, Medicine and Health Care*. 1992;20:7-16.

Reprinted with permission of the American Society of Law & Medicine

Major segments of the news media, as well as many scientific journals, have produced innumerable articles and stories that polarize issues about proper protections for animals involved in research. The prevailing exposition of the issues is the following: On the one hand, animal lovers make emotional appeals to the public's attachment to animals and use clever tactics to increase the vulnerability of universities and institutions of research. On the other hand, arrogant scientists refuse to respond to public controversy, have an inherent conflict of interest in reviewing research involving animals, and are out to advance their careers and interests, callously using animals as means to that end. As a result, journalists warn NIH officials that they "can expect continuing criticism from two disparate and opposing groups—animal welfare activists, who consider NIH the fox guarding the chickens . . . and scientists and administrators from the research community, who regard tighter restrictions as unnecessarily burdensome."

Lost in these somewhat hackneyed ways of polarizing the issues is a set of deep and extremely interesting philosophical problems about the position, if any, that animals used in research should occupy in our moral scheme. The most fundamental problem, in my judgment, is whether animals used in research have any moral standing, and, if so, how that standing should be expressed. . . . While I do not offer a comprehensive resolution of the issues, I do criticize what has become the received view in contemporary philosophical and scientific literature on moral standing.

. . . participants in current discussions about animals are so divided that they do not agree whether the issues are ethical, or even, for that matter, whether they are issues worthy of discussion.

The main problem in contemporary moral theory about animals is that we have not found a compelling account of why we are so special that we deserve moral standing, whereas animals do not; for that matter, we lack a compelling account of why the so-called "higher" animals nonetheless deserve a lower standing than humans do.

As long as one holds out for high-level cognitive criteria on the basis of which humans alone qualify for moral standing, animals will not be viewed as having significant standing. But if one looks not merely to the capacity to experience pain, but to cognitive capacities such as intention, understanding, and belief, animals may come to have protection under these criteria.

In a post-Darwinian period, the fact that we have the same ancestors as the apes provides a powerful reason for holding that we are very much like our evolutionary kin, whatever the differences may be. Evolutionary theory promotes the ideas of continuity and continua, not sharp breaks. If it did not, much research with animals would be pointless. Coming to grips with this fact is a big part of our struggle with the problem of moral standing.

We have before us a series of very tough questions, and no well formed body of answers. Moreover, I believe a more extensive examination of these issues that moves toward consensus will be much tougher to attain than it has been in the area of research with human subjects. These issues are and will remain ticklish and resistant to the formation of a consensus, or any form of agreement. The main, but not sole reason, has to do with our divergent views of moral standing.

■ **DHHS Working Group on the Costs of Research. Management of research costs: indirect costs. Washington, D.C., 1992.**

Indirect costs of research are those expenses that cannot be readily and exclusively identified with research. They are often referred to as overhead and include such expenses as Departmental Administration, General Administration and General Expenses, Sponsored Projects Administration (collectively, Administration); Operations and Maintenance, and Depreciation or Use Allowances (together, Facilities); and Library and Student Services. The Office of Management and Budget (OMB) has established cost principles that govern the determination of which costs are allowable and how they are allocated. Since a 20-percent cap on indirect costs was removed in 1966, the proportion of spending for indirect costs has risen steadily, reaching 46.4 percent of direct costs in 1990.

In October 1991, OMB responded promptly to concerns about inappropriate reimbursement of indirect costs by tightening and clarifying OMB guidelines on unallowable costs and limiting to 26 percent the Administration component of indirect cost rates. This action addresses the indirect cost issue for the short-term. However, long-term issues remain.

The most fundamental issue of the entire public discussion was the need to clarify the basic policy regarding cost reimbursement. The question remains, Should the Federal Government provide full cost reimbursement or a "fair share" of the costs of conducting research? This issue is not explicitly defined in the cost principles, and there are differences of definition and practice among Federal agencies and among partners in the research enterprise.

Using this historical trend data, three projections of average indirect cost rates for the year 2000 were made. The projections were based on trends over the last 10, 5, and 3 years. They indicate that by the year 2000, indirect costs, barring some intervention, would increase by another 5.1 to 7.4 percentage points above the projected 1992 level. Most of the increase would be in Facility costs.

The projections suggest that, without some action to contain this growth, the amount available for direct costs will be reduced.

Several long-term options for improvement to the system for reimbursement of indirect costs are addressed in the following categories: Data, Standardization, Incentives, and Simplification.

This study has demonstrated that the issue of indirect costs can no longer be treated as separate and independent. It must be viewed from the broadest perspective, as it impacts the conduct and support of research. The integrity, comprehension, and uniformity of the indirect cost reimbursement system is essential to continuing public support of research. This report will contribute to the Federal-wide consideration of a number of options across a range of important science policy issues. With this analysis, it now may be possible to more explicitly define specific program and management options and to determine in greater detail the impact of alternative approaches. This effort is not complete. It is expected that the data and policy options articulated here will further enlighten debate and careful Federal action in the interest of a robust United States research enterprise.

■ **Dickens BM. Living tissue and organ donors and property law: more on Moore.** *Journal of Contemporary Health Law and Policy.* **1992;8:73-93.**

Reprinted with permission of *The Journal of Contemporary Health Law and Policy.*

John Moore's claim that his medical mistreatment justified the award of the three billion dollars he sought was likely to attract attention, but the amount of compensation for which he sued was not as extraordinary as the basis of his claim in property law. Moore first visited the University of California's Medical Center at Los Angeles after learning that he had hairy-cell leukemia. . . . he regularly went to UCLA Medical Center from his home in Seattle in order to donate samples of blood, blood serum, skin, bone marrow, and sperm.

Moore stated that while he was under treatment by the defendant physicians, he was advised that the splenectomy and later donations of body substances were required for his health and well-being. He further complained that the physicians concealed both research on his cells and their plans to exploit financially their exclusive access to Moore as derived from the physician-patient relationship.

Moore sued for conversion of his property. He also stated an additional twelve causes of action, namely lack of informed consent, breach of fiduciary duty, fraud and deceit, unjust enrichment, quasi-contract, bad faith breach of the implied covenant of good faith and fair dealing, intentional infliction of emotional distress, negligent misrepresentation, intentional interference with prospective advantageous economic relationships, slander of title, accounting, and declaratory relief.

The majority in *Moore* approached the question of property rights in cells extracted from a living person's body primarily in terms of public or social policy. . . . Nothing in the *Moore* decision suggests that living persons who intend to donate tissues or organs for almost direct transplantation into designated recipients may not invoke their property rights in such materials to advance their own objectives. A body of case law exists that supports this contention. Nonetheless, if this case law is not considered persuasive, then property law should be extended to protect such donors' interests consistently with the reasoning applied in *Moore.*

The speed and scope of biotechnological processing of human cells into therapeutically useful products cannot be reliably predicted, although it is anticipated that tissue and organ donations from living persons will remain significant to therapy. Accordingly, tissue and organ donations will continue to warrant the law's instrumental protection through legal recognition of donors' claims to control the destination and use of their *in vitro* body materials.

■ **Fisher JC. The silicone controversy—when will science prevail?**
N Engl J Med. **1992;326:1696-1698.**

Abstracted from information appearing in *NEJM*. Reprinted with permission of the *New England Journal of Medicine*.

The fate of the silicone-gel breast implant may have been foretold in 1988 when a member of the Food and Drug Administration's advisory panel on general and plastic surgical devices suggested that because the benefits of breast implants were unclear, their use should not be allowed if there was any associated risk. Several members of the advisory panel and the FDA have recently displayed similar insensitivity to the demonstrated needs of more than a million women who since 1963 have sought breast implantation for cosmetic or reconstructive purposes.

The attitude of the FDA and its actions this past year have depended largely on the exaggerated claims of consumer-advocacy groups and on poorly documented assertions. And there are indications that the FDA's approach will extend to other silicone medical products as well.

Meanwhile, the carefully considered position statements of many respected organizations . . . seem to have been ignored by the FDA. These and other responsible professional organizations have sought to place the risks of silicone implantation in perspective with respect to the benefits derived, but with little success.

One reason why we do not know more about the durability of implants is because failure has been uncommon, and in the absence of reliable imaging methods, surgical exploration of asymptomatic women cannot be justified.

The worries prompted by the efforts of Public Citizen, the FDA, and the press have caused many patients without symptoms to ask that their implants be removed or exchanged, a process that offers some opportunity to define the rate of implant failure. But reports of failure are influenced by new variables that confound interpretation.

Only two manufacturers of silicone breast implants remain in the American market. Expansion and development have moved to Europe, where review of the same evidence has produced conclusions contrary to those of the FDA.

But the impact of the FDA's current position will be harshest on women who for their own reasons want breast reconstruction or cosmetic surgery in the future and who will now be subject to the agency's complex guidelines.

■ **Foreman Jr CH. The fast track: federal agencies and the political demand for AIDS drugs.** *Brookings Review.* **1991;9:31-37.**

Reprinted with permission of The Brookings Institution.

One central challenge posed by the HIV epidemic has been the quest for faster bureaucratic action. In particular, AIDS has generated substantial pressure to speed the availability of treatments and vaccines. Increased congressional funding has been one, but not the only, issue. Faster results require that the agencies receiving the money use it in ways that successfully hasten a variety of processes. . . . In their response to the AIDS crisis, the National Institutes of Health and the Food and Drug Administration have dramatically and distinctively transformed their structures and processes. But the new drugs that are the object of the reforms have been slow to materialize. And there is no reason to expect this state of affairs to change soon.

Demands for haste in making available AIDS drugs have concentrated on three areas of concern. First, could the NIH, the nation's primary custodian of basic biomedical research, sort through competing research ideas faster, getting the money to researchers without delay? Second, could the NIH and the FDA speed the discovery and clinical evaluation of potential vaccines and treatments for AIDS? And third, could the FDA, responsible for policing the safety and effectiveness of pharmaceutical products, "grease the skids" of the regulatory process, leading to faster approval for distribution of AIDS-related medications?

Despite the change in process it required, the NIH and the FDA embraced fast tracking for AIDS because faster processing promised a concrete, plausible response to the epidemic. The real trick was to make haste in ways that did not unacceptably threaten the agencies' basic identities or compromise their core missions.

The biggest frustration in trying to speed the availability of vaccines and treatments for AIDS is that the policy tools available (more money, more scientists involved in the search, greater coordination, faster dissemination of research results) cannot guarantee success.

. . . AIDS (and especially AIDS advocacy) has clearly led to considerable changes in institutional structure, procedure, and mindset, at least for this one disease.

AIDS advocates have effectively challenged the establishment, both at the top in policy debates, and from below, through an insurgent movement toward "community-based" research that makes treatment available to as many people as possible.

In recent years various government officials and disease advocates have allied with supporters of regulatory relief for drug manufacturers to help propel three important reforms. One is expedited review . . . of medications for life-threatening or severely debilitating illnesses.

The second reform is the so-called treatment IND, through which an Investigational New Drug . . . may be distributed to limited populations.

A third and related reform . . . is the so-called "parallel track" policy that . . . would make promising new drugs available "through studies without concurrent control groups to monitor drug safety that are conducted in parallel with the principal controlled clinical investigations."

The NIH and the FDA have embraced ideas for speedier drug review and patient access that probably only a handful of desperate patients, business representatives, and efficiency-crazed academics would have supported a decade ago.

■ Kessler DA. The basis of the FDA's decision on breast implants. *N Engl J Med.* **1992;326:1713-1715.**

Abstracted from information appearing in *NEJM*. Reprinted with permission of the *New England Journal of Medicine*.

On April 16, 1992, the Food and Drug Administration announced that breast implants filled with silicone gel would be available only through controlled clinical studies and that women who need such implants for breast reconstruction would be assured of access to these studies.

Although the decision to limit access to breast implants was in step with the recommendations of an FDA advisory panel, it was one of the most controversial decisions ever made by the agency. It has left the FDA open to criticism on both flanks: from those who argue that the FDA should not let any women have breast implants as long as their safety and effectiveness have not been demonstrated, and from those who argue that women ought to be free to weigh the known risks against the personal benefits of an implant and make an independent choice about whether to have one.

The FDA was established as a result of a social mandate. Caveat emptor has never been—and will never be—the philosophy at the FDA. Manufacturers have vested interests. Between those interests and the interests of patients, the FDA must be the arbiter. To argue that people ought to be able to choose their own risks, that government should not intervene, even in the face of inadequate information, is to impose an unrealistic burden on people when they are most vulnerable to manufacturers' assertions: when they are desperately ill, when they are hoping against hope for a cure, or when they are seeking to enhance their physical appearance. Those are precisely the situations in which the legal and ethical justification for the FDA's existence is greatest, however. The decision about breast implants reflects that need.

. . . . Had the FDA failed to intervene, the uncontrolled and widespread availability of breast implants would probably have continued for another 30 years—without producing any meaningful clinical data about their safety and effectiveness. Such a situation is obviously unacceptable. Once and for all, we need to gather information about the safety and effectiveness of these medical devices that have been so widely used for so many years.

■ Kirschstein RL. Research on women's health. *American Journal of Public Health.* **1991;81:291-293.**

Reprinted with permission of the American Public Health Association.

The Office of Research on Women's Health of the National Institutes of Health (NIH) was established in September 1990 to strengthen and enhance the efforts of the NIH to improve the prevention, diagnosis, and treatment of illness in women and to enhance research related to diseases and conditions that affect women.

While the new NIH unit is entitled "Office of *Research* on Women's Health," the concerns in the community are about a much greater series of issues than *research.*

Clearly, there is a deep frustration out there which a *research* unit alone cannot hope to change but which the Office of Research on Women's Health will address. It will attempt to bring changes in the system by setting up a series of studies and conferences to better articulate what the research agenda on women's health issues should be as the United States enters the 21st century. In addition, the Office will try to work with women's advocacy groups to develop a better set of issues related to areas of research.

■ Nelson JL. Transplantation through a glass darkly. *Hastings Center Report.* **1992;22:6-8.**

Bioethical problems take many different forms, and fascinate many different kinds of people.

But there seem to be only two kinds of bioethical problems that typically pull into their orbits not only theorists and practitioners, but pickets and protesters as well. When it comes to the treatment of fetuses and animals, people take to the streets. On the same day that demonstrators on both sides of the abortion issue lamented the Supreme Court's decision in *Casey,* representatives of PETA (People for the Ethical Treatment of Animals) gathered at the University of Pittsburgh to protest the implantation of a baboon's liver in a thirty-five-year-old man—the father of two children—whose own liver had been destroyed by hepatitis B virus.

Here I try to pull moral consideration of nonhumans closer to the ethical center, arguing that thinking about the fate of nonhumans at our hands shares with abortion—indeed, with many of our culture's most difficult moral issues—a fundamental problem: we don't really know what we are talking about. More concretely, we're at a loss to say what it is about baboons that makes their livers fair game, when we wouldn't dare take vital organs from those of our own species whose abilities to live rich, full lives are no greater than those of the nonhumans we seem so willing to prey upon. Unless we're able to isolate and defend the relevant moral distinction, we should reject the seductive image of solving the problem of organ shortage by maintaining colonies of animals at the ready for transplantation on demand.

Cross-species transplantation crystallizes a certain kind of moral conflict between humans and other animals . . .

There are numerous ways in which we might strive to save and enhance lives, including many that are more efficient than killing animals who resemble us in no small degree—ways that do not burden us by reinforcing our commitment to moral positions we do not fully understand, and may not be able to maintain.

We ought to drop xenograft research and therapy, investing the resources of human effort, ingenuity, and money it consumes elsewhere. We don't now know what the judgment of history regarding our relationship with nonhumans will be, but there's no reason to be sanguine about it. What this uncertainty says for our overall relationship with animals may still be a matter for debate, but there's no compelling need to make matters any worse.

■ **Office of Research on Women's Health.** *Report of the National Institutes of Health: Opportunities for Research on Women's Health.* **Bethesda, Md.: National Institutes of Health, 1992. NIH Publication No. 92-3457.**

At the end of the 1980s, irrefutable national data and statistics pointed to a crisis in women's health: a crisis that has stunned citizens, policymakers, and the biomedical community.

The startling realization is that most of the biomedical knowledge about the causes, expression, and treatment of these diseases derives from studies of men and is applied to women with the supposition that there are no differences. . . . As the statistics on death and disease specific to women were integrated and interpreted, concerned individuals became acutely aware that health problems specific to women are worsening and that we currently do not have all the knowledge necessary to reverse this trend.

To focus the biomedical research community on these issues of women's health and to garner their knowledge into a comprehensive plan about how to systematically and expeditiously address those issues, the Office of Research on Women's Health sponsored the Workshop on Opportunities for Research on Women's Health. The goal of both this workshop and the series of events preceding it was to develop a comprehensive research agenda to investigate women's health issues.

As health needs become more widespread in the Nation and funding becomes less available, the goal of solving the health problems facing women must be considered in the design of biomedical research studies. Solving a health problem entails a four-step process (these steps may be simultaneous): recognition, response, research, and reversal.

Scientists, practitioners, patients, and the public, of both genders, must be sensitized about the need, value, and benefits of such directed research and treatment. The research agenda for women's health issues is a vehicle for addressing past gender inequalities and, hopefully, for guiding undertakings by other Federal agencies, academic institutions, pharmaceutical manufacturers, and public and private sector agencies and organizations.

■ Pardes H, West A, Pincus HA. Physicians and the animal-rights movement. *N Engl J Med.* 1991;324:1640-1643.

Abstracted from information appearing in *NEJM*. Reprinted with permission of the *New England Journal of Medicine*.

The current animal-rights movement threatens the future of health science far more than many physicians recognize. The movement is no fringe group of fanatics who cannot have a serious effect on the real world. It is led by politically shrewd people who have built a powerful machine opposed to all animal studies in the life sciences. By impugning the motives of scientists, inaccurately portraying the conditions under which most animal research takes place, and often camouflaging the radical nature of their true goal, the movement's leaders have won support from many well-meaning but misguided sympathizers with animal welfare. The cost to human welfare could be vast.

Biomedical institutions across the country are under assault. It is crucial that physicians help keep medical science alive by informing people both about the reality of research using animals and about a problem that is on its way to becoming a crisis.

It is a critical part of the medical-research community's job to define optimal animal care in the most scrupulously humane terms. It is critical to make rigorous schooling in such care a part of all training programs. It is critical to be vigilant in ensuring that scientists comply with regulations and that if a failure occurs, it is identified and corrections are made immediately. Efforts to achieve these ends have been growing in intensity and must continue to do so.

It is also critical that clinicians help to preserve medical progress, to protect their colleagues in the laboratory and the future lives of patients, by counterbalancing the extremist actions and statements of animal-rights groups.

Victories for the animal-rights movement may be steps in the direction of eliminating animal studies regardless of the cost to human beings. Nevertheless, perhaps the greatest danger to animal research (and its potential benefits) "is not the activity of its opponents, but the inactivity of its defenders."

Having seen the lives of the sick and their families savaged by illness, doctors must help prevent ideology from blocking medical progress. What individual members of the medical community do now could be crucial to a great many patients in the future.

■ **United States General Accounting Office.** *Federal Research: System for Reimbursing Universities' Indirect Costs Should Be Reevaluated.* **Washington, D.C.: United States General Accounting Office, 1992.**

For every dollar spent for federally funded university research, subject to certain exclusions, the government now pays an average of about 50 cents more to cover its share of university overhead, or indirect costs. Concerned about escalating indirect cost rates and the appropriateness of individual charges covered by the rates, the Chairman, Subcommittee on Oversight and Investigations, House Committee on Energy and Commerce, asked GAO to identify inappropriate indirect costs charged to the government, the causes of the inappropriate charges, and the corrective actions being taken. Because of the significant problems identified in the indirect cost reimbursement system, GAO also identified alternative ways for approaching the reimbursement process at universities in the future.

Because of inadequate federal guidance and oversight and weak internal controls at the universities, the government has been charged millions of dollars for unallowable, questionable, or improperly allocated indirect costs. These charges include unallowable costs, such as entertainment and foreign travel unrelated to research, as well as overallocations of otherwise allowable costs, such as utility and depreciation costs.

GAO believes the depth and persistence of the problems and the upward trend in indirect charges over the years make this an opportune time to consider fundamental changes to the existing reimbursement system. A multiagency task force, led by OMB, is addressing the need for such changes. . . . GAO believes that OMB needs to involve the university community in examining possible approaches for restructuring the system.

To assist this process, GAO has identified and analyzed a number of alternative approaches, including their advantages and disadvantages, that it believes should be considered in making structural changes to the reimbursement system. Some of the alternatives, such as instituting a uniform flat rate or different flat rates for different categories of universities, offer greater opportunities to simplify the system than others. Although GAO is not recommending a specific alternative or set of alternatives, it believes the ultimate objective should be to establish a system that sets some reasonable limit on the amount of indirect costs the government would reimburse; it is administratively efficient for both the government and the universities; and protects the government's interest by providing for sufficient controls, audits, and periodic analysis.

Regardless of any long-term solution that is selected, GAO believes it is inefficient to have two federal agencies administering the program, particularly when they are using fundamentally different approaches.

GAO recommends that the Director, OMB, designate a single cognizant federal agency, using a consistent approach, to negotiate indirect cost rates for federally sponsored research at universities. GAO further recommends that OMB examine ways to more directly involve a cross section of the university community in the work of the task force, either through direct membership or a separate advisory committee, in evaluating alternative methods (including, but not limited to, ones that GAO has identified) for reimbursing universities for indirect costs related to federally sponsored research.

■ Vawter DE, Caplan A. Strange brew: the politics and ethics of fetal tissue transplant research in the United States. *Journal of Laboratory and Clinical Medicine.* 1992;120:30-34.

Reprinted with permission from Mosby-Year Book, Inc.

A great deal of concern has been expressed during the past few years about the ethics of using fetal tissue in biomedical research. The debate about the morality of such research has been especially heated in the United States. Yet research using fetal tissue, even for the purpose of transplantation, is not new.

Four major objections have been raised against the transplantation of tissue from electively aborted fetuses. Only the first and second of these have played a role in the public policy debate in the United States about the existing moratorium on the funding of fetal tissue transplantation research.

1. Abortion is so immoral that any use of the tissue is immoral as well.
2. The transplantation of fetal tissue will alter abortion practices in ways that will make the use of fetal tissue immoral.

3. The transplantation of fetal tissue into patients is premature.

4. The transplantation of fetal tissue is contrary to the interests of women.

The central premise underlying both the ban on federal funding and the certification requirement in the legislation in the House of Representatives is that women will have abortions they would not otherwise have in order to donate fetal tissue to anonymous others.

No empirical evidence exists that women would abort to donate fetal tissue to assist anonymous others.

The current ban on federal funding of fetal tissue transplantation research rests on a set of fallacious assumptions. The only way of explaining the persistence of a public policy that rests on patently false empirical foundations is in terms of politics, not ethics.

Jay Stein

A lthough the 20th century has seen unprecedented breakthroughs in health care, there are still millions of people suffering from diseases that have no cure. The imminent research opportunities that we face are threatened by several controversial social and political issues. Three of these issues directly affect the fundamental process of research and medical education in our academic health centers. Animal research, fetal tissue research, and indirect costs not only raise interesting questions regarding public policy, but also raise furor within many diverse groups. Such controversy threatens to thwart medical research and the hope that such research instills in individuals suffering from diseases such as Alzheimer's, Parkinson's, and diabetes. My perspective in commenting on these three issues emanates from my previous experiences as a researcher, educator, and physician, and currently as Provost of the University of Oklahoma Health Sciences Center.

In spite of the extraordinary polarity that animal research engenders, there is absolutely no question in my mind that using animals for medical research is highly justified. The inherent differences in human and animal life are a part of this justification, but most important is the necessity of using animals to achieve a basic understanding of and treatment for various diseases. Over the past century, nearly every medical advancement—from developing a vaccine for polio to the cardiac bypass procedure—has been a result of research done with animals.

There is no substitute for the use of animals in medical research. Many types of in vitro techniques have contributed to biological and medical research but are only supporting mechanisms for the intricate verification process that is necessary. Neither computer or mathematical models, cell or tissue cultures can replicate the complex and mysterious interactions that exist in the complex life system of an animal.

Within this philosophy is a deep concern for the welfare of animals and the humane and kind treatment of them. Public policy has addressed this concern, and today's federal regulations and local enforcement of laboratory standards ensure the well-being of animals used in research. Further regulation will only stymie the research that is critical to reducing suffering and death.

A second issue that threatens to block vital research and potential treatment concerns the use of fetal tissue in research and transplantation. Again, I perceive such research as not only justified, but as critical to the future of medicine in our world. Similar to the unique environment a whole life system (i.e., an animal) gives to researchers, fetal tissue also offers opportunities for which there is no substitute. Being immunologically immature, fetal tissue can be compatibly used as grafts with mature tissue. Unlike adult cells, fetal neurological tissue cells divide rapidly in embryogenesis. Fetal tissue, therefore, offers avenues to treat neurologic diseases that otherwise do not exist.

The opposition to such research is based on fear and irrationality and does not address the true crisis: disease continues to plague human beings. Legislation during the Bush Administration effectively halted federal funding of all human fetal tissue transplantion research. This ban was based on fear that supporting fetal tissue research would imply that the federal government condones abortion. It is unfortunate that politics took precedence over the medical reality: such research was leading scientists to discovering effective treatments of genetic disorders and neurological diseases. The issue of fetal tissue research must be kept separate from the abortion debate.

With the Clinton Administration come new perspectives and direction regarding this issue. Clinton has lifted the ban on funding for fetal tissue research. Guidelines governing the practice of such research are intended to ensure that tissue donation for research and transplantation is kept separate from a woman's decision to have an abortion. The House and Senate, as well as a National Institutes of Health advisory panel, agree on necessary guidelines such as forbidding financial incentives for donating tissue and requiring that a woman's consent for an abortion must be given before consent to donate tissue. As the practice policy becomes finalized, we must not allow "right to life" politics to threaten the opportunities of life-saving discoveries that fetal tissue research promises.

Lastly, we need to address the hot topic of indirect cost reimbursement. Academic health centers across the nation are facing the harsh reality of a new indirect cost reimbursement system that will significantly change dollars recovered from this process.

The Office of Management and Budget's suggested capping of indirect costs at 26% is not the solution to the problem. The purpose of indirect cost recovery is to reimburse the university for expenses incurred by carrying out research for the federal government. Therefore, indirect costs are a part of the overall budget of the university. Capping this cost at such a low level severely affects not only the research of the university but also the education and service programs. The issue is essentially an accounting phenomenon that must be reanalyzed. A reconsideration of allowable expenses and a process to tighten up accounting procedures to estimate the base from which a cap is applied are necessary. While there have been some abuses of this system in the past, this is no reason to put the ax to the budget of the research-oriented institutions in an arbitrary and rigid fashion.

From this very brief review, one can see that the "ivory tower" has no barricades. Academic health centers are susceptible to the same political pressures as any other entity that receives federal and/or state support. Politics are an integral part of our lives and must be considered. The leadership of academic health centers has spent much time in the last decade dealing with issues such as the role of animal research, the appropriateness of fetal tissue research, and the proper way to allocate indirect costs to a given institution. These are only a few examples of a number of public issues that we must be informed about and prepared to come forth to defend and facilitate with the general public.

James A. Zimble

The 13 thought-provoking articles contained in this chapter fully qualify as candidates for controversial and emerging issues. They address matters involving fields of biomedical research that are generating significant controversy today. Although covering widely dissimilar subject matter from property rights of tissue and organ donors to a methodology for determining the indirect costs of research, a common focus is morality and ethics in our pursuit of knowledge.

It has been said that for every issue, no matter how complex or perplexing, there is a simple solution . . . and that solution is invariably wrong! That notion is especially relevant when attempting to deal with societal beliefs about the right or wrong of scientific practices. It has been difficult for our society to articulate a clear definition of scientific ethical or moral behavior either through public policy established by regulation, legislation, or jurisprudence. Even more challenging, of course, is achieving a consensus in our heterogeneous society of individuals who hold widely divergent views of virtuous endeavor. When new discoveries and technology create dilemmas that have never seriously been considered or evaluated, such a problem may be exacerbated.

Nelson states the "fundamental problem" quite well in his provocative article, "Transplantation Through a Glass Darkly." "We really don't know what we are talking about," he says. In the three articles dealing with animal research, we quickly become enmeshed in the moral debate between animal rights vs. the quest for the health and welfare of humankind. Perhaps rather than think of ourselves as beings separate and detached from the natural order and subject to a higher moral law due to our cognition and autonomy, we should accept our role as a part of nature. We need to recognize that our enviable current status at the head of the phylogenetic queue conveys the power and opportunity to exploit the "lesser species," but also carries with it responsibility for our environment.

The articles do not provide an answer to the argument of whether or not we are "right" to exploit animals for our benefit. Instead, they effectively describe the interplay between opportunity and responsibility. We are endowed with an empathy that allows us to perceive the pain and suffering in animals and demands that we continually reassess our rationale for their sacrifice and assiduously seek to eliminate their suffering. As physicians and scientists we are accountable for ensuring humane treatment and avoiding unwarranted pain and death of all those creatures in our custody. We are neither apes nor angels; rather we are the current custodians of our environment, and we need to be compassionate and generous in that role.

The issue of property rights of our tissues, whether for financial compensation or for the privilege of parenting, is examined in the articles by Dickens and Annas. It is extremely difficult to develop public policy that can address complex questions such as rewarding the donor-patient for providing, as a result of therapy, the raw material for the development of intellectual property effected through the ingenuity of the attending physician-researcher. Neither is it easy, even for Solomon, to justly resolve the argument of genetic maternity vs. gestational motherhood. These issues, as well as countless others associated with current and future advances in biomedical technology, can only be made on an individualized basis. These articles aptly explore the many facets of the conflict of ownership. Understanding the lessons of the experiences and judgments described should assist in better preparation of patients, physicians, and researchers. Appropriate informed counseling and anticipation of potential controversy might then lead to the development of policies and procedures that effectively mitigate undesirable outcomes of an exploding biomedical science.

The articles concerning research on women's health very succinctly demonstrate a gender bias in scientific research and a regrettable inattention in the health science community to the biologic differences between males and females. Indeed, the biomedical research designed to enhance the health and well-being of "man" has apparently made "woman" the forgotten gender. Public policy concerning this issue has been effected through regulations of the National Institutes of Health (NIH) in guidance for grants and contracts and in research initiatives seeking to increase study of women's health issues. Such guidance should be successful in directing appropriate attention towards women's health research so that the appalling gaps in health care outcomes between the sexes displayed in the NIH report: *Opportunities for Research on Women's Health* can be effectively closed.

The United States General Accounting Office (GAO) may have afforded those institutions pursuing biomedical research the chance to harness the runaway costs of doing the business of scientific research. The GAO report offers several recommendations to simplify the process of establishing rates for indirect costs as well as leveling the playing field for obtaining federal grants. Hopefully, the task force formed by the Office of Management and Budget to explore that process is prudent enough to recognize the lack of a "customer" presence, as noted in the GAO report. The need for an equitable policy that demands accountability and fiduciary use of taxpayers' dollars and that ensures adequate resources for appropriate biomedical research is obvious. Such policy can best be determined with both payers and players at the table.

The controversies regarding fast-track drug investigation, fetal tissue research, and the silicone breast implant debate are especially thought-provoking with regard to the role of federal agencies in policymaking. Should regulatory agencies such as the Food and Drug Administration serve as surrogate parents for a medically unsophisticated society by proscribing and dictating practices? Or should such agencies serve to set appropriate standards and to educate and caution the public? Should policies articulated by the Secretary of Health and Human Services be dictated by political persuasion or should they be developed by informed counsel? Ineffective, obstructive and arbitrary policy results when policymakers do not properly assess scientific data and when they ignore their customers. Innovative research designed to address the needs of the public is strangled when public policy is made from the top down without listening to the voice of the public.

As we ride this ever-faster rocket of burgeoning biomedical scientific knowledge and technology we can expect an ever-expanding number of new challenges to our societal norms that will tax our public conscience. A collection of articles similar to that offered here provides the ideal forum for meaningful contemplation of the controversies that emerge from these challenges. Finally, such a forum will enable us to start to resolve these problems through the development of effective public policy.

Bibliography

Science, Technology, and Societal Goals

Bondi H. Bridging the gulf. *Technology in Society.* 1992;14:9-14.

Branscomb LM. Does America need a technology policy? *Harvard Business Review.* 1992;70:24-28.

Carnegie Commission on Science, Technology, and Government. *Enabling the Future: Linking Science and Technology to Societal Goals.* Washington, D.C.: Carnegie Commission on Science, Technology, and Government, 1992.

Cassman M. The evolution of a science advisory body in the federal government. *Perspectives in Biology and Medicine.* 1991;34:439-462.

Curlin JW. Science and technology under constitutional separation of powers. *Technology in Society.* 1992;14:63-73.

Newby H. One society, one Wissenschaft: a 21st century vision. *Science and Public Policy.* 1992;19:7-14.

Owen D. Improving the input of scientific advice into political decision making. *Technology in Society.* 1992;14:37-47.

Task Force on the Health of Research. *Chairman's Report to the Committee on Science, Space, and Technology, U.S. House of Representatives, One Hundred Second Congress.* Washington, D.C.: U.S. Government Printing Office, 1992.

Setting Priorities and Allocating Funds for Biomedical Research

Brennan TA. Government and science: stimulation or inhibition. *Bull NY Acad Med.* 1992;68:151-161.

Friedman H. Big science vs. little science: the controversy mounts. *Cosmos.* 1991;1:8-14.

Institute of Medicine. *Research and Service Programs in the PHS: Challenges in Organization.* Washington, D.C.: National Academy Press, 1991.

Kirschner M. The need for unity in the biomedical research community. *Academic Medicine*. 1991;66:577-582.

National Institutes of Health. The "Strategic Plan": mixing salesmanship and science. *The Journal of NIH Research*. 1992;4:33-40.

National Institutes of Health. *The Status of Biomedical Research Facilities: 1990*. Washington, D.C.: U.S. Department of Health and Human Services, 1991.

National Institutes of Health. *Framework for Discussion of Strategies for NIH*. Washington, D.C.: U.S. Department of Health and Human Services, 1992.

Office of Technology Assessment. *Federally Funded Research: Decisions for a Decade*. Washington, D.C.: U.S. Government Printing Office, 1992.

Pardes H. Assessing the past and planning the future to ensure support for biomedical research. *Academic Medicine*. 1991;66:582-584.

Pavitt K. What makes basic research economically useful? *Research Policy*. 1991;20:109-119.

President's Council of Advisors on Science and Technology. *Renewing the Promise: Research-Intensive Universities and the Nation*. Washington, D.C.: United States Government Printing Office, 1992.

Senker J. Evaluating the funding of strategic science: some lessons from British experience. *Research Policy*. 1991;20:29-43.

Sherman JF. Shaping national science policy: some lessons learned. *Academic Medicine*. 1991;66:66-70.

Tauber AI, Sarkar S. The Human Genome Project: has blind reductionism gone too far? *Perspectives in Biology and Medicine*. 1992;35:220-235.

Yager T, Nickerson D, Hood L. The Human Genome Project: creating an infrastructure for biology and medicine. *Trends in Biochemical Sciences*. 1991;16:454-461.

Biotechnology, Biomedical Research, and Global Competition

Burton DF. A new model for U.S. innovation. *Issues in Science and Technology*. 1992;8:52-59.

Davis EB, Weiner JL, Farber NJ, Boyer EG, Robinson EJ. Watching the biotech window of opportunity. *J of Amer Health Policy.* 1992;2:52-55.

Office of Technology Assessment. *Biotechnology in a global economy.* Washington, D.C.: Office of Technology Assessment, 1992.

Vaughan C, Smith BL, Porter RJ. U.S. biomedical science and technology. *Knowledge: Creation, Diffusion, Utilization.* 1992;14:91-109.

Innovative Alliances and Commercial Ventures

Adler RG. Genome research: fulfilling the public's expectations for knowledge and commercialization. *Science.* 1992;257:908-914.

Armstrong JA. University research: new goals, new practices. *Issues in Science and Technology.* 1992-93;IX:50-53.

Blumenthal D. Academic-industry relationships in the life sciences. *JAMA.* 1992;268:3344-3349.

Committee on Government Operations. *Is Science for Sale? Transferring Technology from Universities to Foreign Corporations.* Washington, D.C.: U.S. Government Printing Office, 1992.

Cuatrecasas P. Industry–university alliances in biomedical research. *J Clin Pharmacol.* 1992;32:100-106.

Eisenberg RS. Genes, patents, and product development. *Science.* 1992;257:903-908.

Fishbein EA. Ownership of research data. *Academic Medicine.* 1991;66:129-133.

Healy B. Special report on gene patenting. *New Engl J Med.* 1992;327:664-668.

Kiley TD. Patents on random complementary DNA fragments? *Science.* 1992;257:915-918.

Mansfield E. Academic research and industrial innovation. *Research Policy.* 1991;20:1-12.

Moriarty CM, Purdy JB. University research: planning for the 1990s. *Educational Record.* 1992;Summer:51-56.

Mowery DC. The U.S. national innovation system: origins and prospects for change. *Research Policy.* 1992;21:125-144.

Rosenberg N. Scientific instrumentation and university research. *Research Policy*. 1992;21:381-390.

United States General Accounting Office. *University Research: Controlling Inappropriate Access to Federally Funded Research Results*. Washington, D.C.: United States General Accounting Office, 1992.

Integrity in Scientific Research

Institute of Medicine. *Responsible Science: Ensuring the Integrity of the Research Process*, Volume I. Washington, D.C.: National Academy Press, 1992:1-16.

Maechling C. The laboratory is not a courtroom. *Issues in Science & Technology*. 1992;8:73-77.

Pellegrino ED. Character and the ethical conduct of research. *Accountability in Research*. 1992;2:1-11.

Shimm DS, Spece RG. Industry reimbursement for entering patients into clinical trials: legal and ethical issues. *Annals of Internal Medicine*. 1991;115:148-151.

Ethical Standards for Scientific Publications

Bero LA, Galbraith A, Rennie D. The publication of sponsored symposiums in medical journals. *N Engl J Med*. 1992;327:1135-1140.

Dickersin K, Min YI, Meinert CL. Factors influencing publication of research results. *JAMA*. 1992;267:374-378.

Hillman AL, Eisenberg JM, Pauly MV, et al. Avoiding bias in the conduct and reporting of cost-effectiveness research sponsored by pharmaceutical companies. *N Engl J Med*. 1991;324:1362-1365.

Koren G, Klein N. Bias against negative studies in newspaper reports of medical research. *JAMA*. 1991;266:1824-1826.

Rennie D, Flanagin A, Glass RM. Conflicts of interest in the publication of science. *JAMA*. 1991;266:266-267.

Safer DJ, Krager JM. Effect of a media blitz and a threatened lawsuit on stimulant treatment. *JAMA*. 1992;268:1004-1007.

Wilkes MS, Doblin BH, Shapiro MF. Pharmaceutical advertisements in leading medical journals: experts' assessments. *Annals of Internal Medicine.* 1992;116:912-919.

Public Perceptions of Science: Dilemmas for Policymaking

Institute of Medicine. *Biomedical Politics.* Hanna KE, ed. Washington, D.C.: National Academy Press, 1991.

Jasanoff S. Does public understanding influence public policy? *Chemistry & Industry.* 1991;15:537-540.

Silverstone R. Communicating science to the public. *Science, Technology, & Human Values.* 1991;16:106-110.

Veatch RM. Consensus of expertise: the role of consensus of experts in formulating public policy and estimating facts. *J Med Philos.* 1991;16:427-445.

Wynne B. Knowledges in context. *Science, Technology, & Human Values.* 1991;16:111-121.

Wynne B. Public perception and communication of risks: what do we know? *The Journal of NIH Research.* 1991;3:65-70.

Ziman J. Public understanding of science. *Science, Technology, & Human Values* 1991;16:99-105.

Human Subjects: Protection, Policies, and Practice

Annas GJ. Changing the consent rules for Desert Storm. *N Engl J Med.* 1992;326:770-773.

Brett A, Grodin M. Ethical aspects of human experimentation in health services research. *JAMA.* 1991;265:1854-1857.

Capron AM. Protection of research subjects: do special rules apply in epidemiology? *Law, Medicine, and Health Care.* 1991;44:184-190.

Christakis NA, Panner MJ. Existing international ethical guidelines for human subjects research: some open questions. *Law, Medicine and Health Care.* 1991;19:214-220.

DeGregorio MW. Is tamoxifen chemoprevention worth the risk in healthy women? *The Journal of NIH Research.* 1992;4:84-87.

Dickens B. Issues in preparing ethical guidelines for epidemiological studies. *Law, Medicine and Health Care.* 1991;19:175-183.

Dresser R. Wanted: single, white male for medical research. *Hastings Center Report.* 1992;22:24-29.

Gostin L. Ethical principles for the conduct of human subject research: population-based research and ethics. *Law, Medicine, and Health Care.* 1991;19:191-201.

Hellman S, Hellman DS. Of mice but not men: problems of the randomized clinical trial. *N Engl J Med.* 1991;324:1585-1589.

Ijsselmuiden CB, Faden RR. Research and informed consent in Africa—another look. *N Engl J Med.* 1992;326:830-834.

Osborne NG, Feit MD. The use of race in medical research. *JAMA.* 1992;267:275-279.

Passamani E. Clinical trials—are they ethical? *N Engl J Med.* 1991;324:1589-1592.

Twenty years after: the legacy of the Tuskegee syphilis study. *Hastings Center Report.* 1992;22-29-32.

- Caplan AL. When evil intrudes. *Hastings Center Report.* 1992; 22:29-32.
- Edgar H. Outside the community. *Hastings Center Report.* 1992;22:32-35.
- King PA. The dangers of difference. *Hastings Center Report.* 1992;22:35-38.
- Jones JH. The Tuskegee legacy: AIDS and the black community. *Hastings Center Report.* 1992;22:38-40.

Ethical Challenges in the Use of Genetic Information

Annas GJ. Setting standards for the use of DNA-typing results in the courtroom—the state of the art. *N Engl J Med.* 1992;326:1641-1644.

Council on Ethical and Judicial Affairs, American Medical Association. Use of genetic testing by employers. *JAMA.* 1991;266:1827-1830.

Fletcher JC, Anderson WF. Germ-line gene therapy: a new stage of debate. *Law, Medicine and Health Care.* 1992;20:26-39.

Gostin L. Genetic discrimination: the use of genetically based diagnostic and prognostic tests by employers and insurers. *American J of Law and Med.* 1991;17:109-144.

Juengst ET. Priorities in professional ethics and social policy for human genetics. *JAMA.* 1991;266:1835-1836.

Murray TH. Ethical issues in human genome research. *FASEB J.* 1991;5:55-60.

National Research Council. *DNA Technology in Forensic Science.* Washington, D.C.: National Academy Press; 1992.

Nelkin D, Tancredi L. Classify and control: genetic information in the schools. *American J of Law and Med.* 1991;17:51-73.

Roberts RJ. The societal impact of DNA fingerprint data. *Accountability in Research.* 1992;2:87-92.

Zimmerman BK. Human germ-line therapy: the case for its development and use. *J Med Philos.* 1991;16:593-612.

Effects of Biomedical Research on Patient Care

Annas GJ. The human genome project as social policy: implications for clinical medicine. *Bulletin of the NY Academy of Medicine.* 1992;68:126-134.

Baum BJ. Has modern biology entered the mouth? The clinical impact of biological research. *Journal of Dental Education.* 1991;55:299-303.

Council on Ethical and Judicial Affairs, American Medical Association. Gender disparities in clinical decision making. *JAMA.* 1991;266:559-562.

Levine C, Stein GL. What's in a name? The policy implications of the CDC definition of AIDS. *Law, Medicine and Health Care.* 1991;19:278-290.

Meyer BR. Biotechnology and therapeutics: expensive treatments and limited resources. A view from the hospital. *Clinical Pharmacology & Therapeutics.* 1992;51:359-365.

Controversial and Emerging Issues

Annas GJ. Using genes to define motherhood—the California solution. *N Engl J Med.* 1992;326:417-420.

Beauchamp TL. The moral standing of animals in medical research. *Law, Medicine and Health Care.* 1992;20:7-16.

DHHS Working Group on the Costs of Research. Management of research costs: indirect costs. Washington, D.C., 1992.

Dickens BM. Living tissue and organ donors and property law: more on *Moore. Journal of Contemporary Health Law and Policy.* 1992;8:73-93.

Fisher JC. The silicone controversy—when will science prevail? *N Engl J Med.* 1992;326:1696-1698.

Foreman Jr CH. The fast track: federal agencies and the political demand for AIDS drugs. *Brookings Review.* 1991;9:31-37.

Kessler DA. The basis of the FDA's decision on breast implants. *N Engl J Med.* 1992;326:1713-1715.

Kirschstein RL. Research on women's health. *American Journal of Public Health.* 1991;81:291-293.

Nelson JL. Transplantation through a glass darkly. *Hastings Center Report.* 1992;22:6-8.

Office of Research on Women's Health. *Report of the National Institutes of Health: Opportunities for Research on Women's Health.* Bethesda, Md.: National Institutes of Health, 1992. NIH Publication No. 92-3457.

Pardes H, West A, Pincus HA. Physicians and the animal-rights movement. *N Engl J Med.* 1991;324:1640-1643.

United States General Accounting Office. *Federal Research: System for Reimbursing Universities' Indirect Costs Should Be Reevaluated.* Washington, D.C.: United States General Accounting Office, 1992.

Vawter DE, Caplan A. Strange brew: the politics and ethics of fetal tissue transplant research in the United States. *Journal of Laboratory and Clinical Medicine.* 1992;120:30-34.